Study Guide

Nursing Care of Children
Principles & Practice

Fourth Edition

Susan Rowen James, PhD, RN
Kristine Ann Nelson, MN, RN
Jean Weiler Ashwill, MSN, RN

Revised by
Julie White, RN, MSN
Adjunct Faculty
Valparaiso University
Valparaiso, Indiana
Director of Education
IU Health La Porte Hospital
La Porte, Indiana

Previous authors
Anne-Marie Kiehne, PhD, RN
Assistant Clinical Professor
College of Health Professions
Temple University
Philadelphia, Pennsylvania

Christine M. Rosner, PhD, RN
Dean and Professor
School of Nursing and Allied Health Professions
Holy Family University
Philadelphia, Pennsylvania

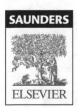

SAUNDERS

ELSEVIER

ELSEVIER
SAUNDERS

3251 Riverport Lane
St. Louis, Missouri 63043

STUDY GUIDE FOR NURSING CARE OF CHILDREN, FOURTH EDITION　　　ISBN: 978-1-4557-0706-5

Notices

Knowledge and best practice in this field are constantly changing. As new research and experience broaden our understanding, changes in research methods, professional practices, or medical treatment may become necessary.

Practitioners and researchers must always rely on their own experience and knowledge in evaluating and using any information, methods, compounds, or experiments described herein. In using such information or methods they should be mindful of their own safety and the safety of others, including parties for whom they have a professional responsibility.

With respect to any drug or pharmaceutical products identified, readers are advised to check the most current information provided (i) on procedures featured or (ii) by the manufacturer of each product to be administered, to verify the recommended dose or formula, the method and duration of administration, and contraindications. It is the responsibility of practitioners, relying on their own experience and knowledge of their patients, to make diagnoses, to determine dosages and the best treatment for each individual patient, and to take all appropriate safety precautions.

To the fullest extent of the law, neither the Publisher nor the authors, contributors, or editors, assume any liability for any injury and/or damage to persons or property as a matter of products liability, negligence or otherwise, or from any use or operation of any methods, products, instructions, or ideas contained in the material herein.

Content Manager: Michele D. Hayden
Content Development Specialist: Heather Bays
Publishing Services Manager: Hemamalini Rajendrababu
Project Manager: Divya Krish
Design Direction: Paula Catalano

Printed in the United States of America

Last digit is the print number:　9　8　7　6　5　4　3　2　1

Working together to grow
libraries in developing countries

www.elsevier.com | www.bookaid.org | www.sabre.org

ELSEVIER　BOOK AID International　Sabre Foundation

Preface

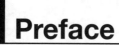

The objective of this Study Guide to accompany James and Ashwill: *Nursing Care of Children: Principles and Practice,* fourth edition, is to facilitate your understanding of the material presented in the textbook.

ORGANIZATION

Each chapter in this Study Guide is meant to be used as a studying tool for its corresponding textbook chapter. Chapters are presented in the same numerical order as in the textbook. At the end of this manual, you will find answers to the Student Learning Exercises and Review Questions for all Study Guide chapters.

FEATURES

Each chapter includes the following features, which are designed to help you better comprehend and organize the textbook material.

1. **Helpful Hints** refer you to other chapters in the core textbook or to other references for background information that may enhance your understanding of the chapter.

2. **Student Learning Exercises** are organized primarily to follow the order of content in the textbook and are also grouped by types of exercises. To emphasize the significant content of each chapter, we have presented questions in a variety of formats—matching, fill in the blank, short answer, true or false, and crossword puzzles. Bold topical headings

corresponding to those in the textbook serve as transitions from one subject to the next. The answers for all these exercises are provided at the back of the Study Guide.

3. **Suggested Learning Activities** are opportunities for you to apply your knowledge to real-life situations, either clinical or personal.

4. **Student Learning Applications** include case studies with accompanying questions that are designed for you to apply your knowledge to hypothetical situations that mirror real-life events in pediatric nursing. In many cases, there may be no single correct answer, and we hope that by sharing your answers with other students, you will broaden your perspective of the clinical situation.

5. **Review Questions** are provided in multiple-choice format to give you an opportunity to review key content quickly. The answers to these questions are also provided at the back of the manual.

It is the intention that the learning activities presented in this Study Guide will help you to apply the content of the textbook directly to the practice of pediatric nursing.

Julie White, RN, MSN
Anne-Marie Kiehne, PhD, RN
Christine M. Rosner, PhD, RN

Contents

1 Introduction to Nursing Care of Children

HELPFUL HINT

A textbook covering the fundamentals of nursing or United States government websites can provide useful supplemental information on many of the topics covered in this chapter.

STUDENT LEARNING EXERCISES

Definitions

Match each term with its definition.

1. _____ Advocacy

2. _____ Bioethics

3. _____ Ethical dilemma

4. _____ Morbidity rate

5. _____ Infant mortality rate

6. _____ Standard of care

7. _____ Standardized practices

a. Level of care expected from a professional
b. Ratio of sick to well people in a defined population
c. Procedures that allow nurses to perform duties that are usually part of the medical practice
d. Speaking or acting in support of a policy or a person's rights
e. Number of deaths per 1000 live births that occur within the first 12 months of life
f. Situation in which no solution seems completely satisfactory
g. Rules or principles that govern ethical conduct related to healthcare

Historical Perspectives

Answer as either true (T) or false (F).

8. _____ Throughout history children have been valued and protected by society.

9. _____ During the nineteenth century, the most serious health problems facing children were directly related to poverty and overcrowding.

10. _____ William Cadogan created the first public health program for mothers and children.

11. _____ Hospital policies have changed in response to an increased awareness of children's emotional and psychological needs.

12. _____ Because of technological advances, children with chronic disabilities are living longer.

13. _____ Title V of the Social Security Act provides funds for maternal-child healthcare programs.

14. _____ Family-centered care views parents and health care professionals as equal partners in children's health care.

15. How has the Association for the Care of Children's Health (ACCH) affected the care of hospitalized children?

_____

_____

Current Trends and Issues

16. What is *Healthy People 2020?* _____

_____

17. What are diagnosis-related groups (DRGs)? _____

_____

18. Define *case management.* _____

_____

19. What are clinical pathways? _____

_____

20. List two public health insurance programs for children.

 a. _____

 b. _____

Describe the following health care assistance programs

21. WIC _____

_____

22. EPSDT _____

_____

23. Public Law 99-457 _____

_____

24. Healthy Start _____

_____

Statistics on Infant and Child Health

Answer as either true (T) or false (F).

25. _____ African-American infants are more likely than white infants to be born prematurely.

26. _____ Poverty plays an important role in infant mortality.

27. _____ The United States has the third lowest infant mortality rate among developed nations.

28. _____ Unintentional injuries are the leading cause of death among children 1 to 19 years of age.

Ethical Perspectives in Child Health Nursing

Match each ethical principle with its correct description.

29. _____ Beneficence

30. _____ Nonmaleficence

31. _____ Autonomy

32. _____ Justice

a. The obligation to avoid causing harm
b. The obligation to treat all people equally and fairly
c. The obligation to do or promote good for others
d. The right of individuals for self-determination

Legal Issues

Answer as either true (T) or false (F).

33. _____ Nurse practice acts do not vary from state to state.

34. _____ Standards of care are set by professional associations and describe the level of care that should be expected from practitioners.

35. _____ Nurses should be familiar with the policies, procedures, and protocols in the institutions in which they work.

36. What are the four elements of negligence?

    a. _____

    b. _____

    c. _____

    d. _____

37. What are the four requirements of informed consent?

    a. _____

    b. _____

    c. _____

    d. _____

Social Issues

Answer as either true (T) or false (F).

38. _____ Children living in poverty are more likely to be in poor health than are children in other socioeconomic groups.

39. _____ The number of families living in poverty is higher in the Southern and Western regions of the United States.

40. _____ Single mothers and children are the fastest growing group of homeless people.

41. _____ Nurses should ask children about whether there is violence in the home, school, and neighborhood.

42. _____ Parents should limit their children's exposure to electronic media (e.g., television, computers, video games) to less than 4 hours a day.

The Professional Nurse

43. List the various roles assumed by the pediatric nurse.

_____

_____

_____

44. How do the roles and responsibilities of a pediatric nurse practitioner differ from those of a clinical nurse specialist?

_____

_____

_____

45. Identify four work settings for pediatric nurses other than acute care.

a. _____

b. _____

c. _____

d. _____

Nursing of Children: The Nursing Process

Match each step of the nursing process with its correct description.

46. _____ Assessment

47. _____ Diagnosis

48. _____ Planning

49. _____ Implementation

50. _____ Evaluation

a. Actual initiation and completion of nursing actions
b. Identification of actual or potential health problems for an individual, family, or community
c. Prioritization of nursing diagnoses and identification of expected outcomes and nursing interventions
d. Examination of nursing intervention results versus the stated expected outcomes
e. Systematic collection of data to determine health status of the child and his or her family

SUGGESTED LEARNING ACTIVITIES

1. Observe a pediatric nurse practitioner or a clinical nurse specialist. What type of education was needed for this advanced practice? What did you find most interesting about your experience?

2. Observe a nurse in a community-based setting. What types of services or care are provided in this setting? What is the nurse's role in this setting? How does the role of the nurse in a community-based setting differ from the role in an acute-care setting?

STUDENT LEARNING APPLICATION

Enhance your learning by discussing the following issues with other students.

1. Share with other students ethical or legal situations you have experienced or read about that involved nurses and pediatric clients. Discuss your thoughts on the outcome of each situation.

2. Search the nursing literature and the Internet for information about health problems facing homeless children. Share your findings with other students.

REVIEW QUESTIONS

Choose the best answer.

1. Which statement about the principles of pediatric nursing is correct?
   a. The core of pediatric nursing is child-focused care.
   b. The role of the nurse as patient advocate is unique to pediatric nursing.
   c. All aspects of a child's care must be tailored to the child's developmental level.
   d. Health education and promotion efforts are directed toward curing illness.

2. Lillian Wald is recognized for which contribution to nursing?
   a. She discouraged the practice of tightly swaddling infants in three layers of clothing.
   b. She initiated public health nursing at the Henry Street Settlement.
   c. She promoted family-centered care for hospitalized children.
   d. She developed infection control procedures in hospitals and foundling homes.

3. Which statement about social issues relating to children's health is true?
   a. Fewer children in the United States are living in poverty.
   b. Violence in the schools is decreasing.
   c. Birth rates among U.S. adolescents are declining.
   d. The number of insured children is increasing.

4. A practice model that uses a systematic approach to identify specific clients and manage their care is:
   a. case management.
   b. the nursing process.
   c. a clinical pathway.
   d. a health maintenance organization.

5. During the assessment phase of the nursing process, the nurse:
   a. collects data, groups findings, and writes nursing diagnoses.
   b. prioritizes nursing diagnoses and identifies expected orders and nursing interventions.
   c. initiates nursing interventions and documents the response of the child and his or her family.
   d. determines whether the child or child's family have made progress.

6. Which is a requirement for informed consent?
   a. A child who understands an explanation may give consent for treatment.
   b. It is not necessary to determine whether a parent understands an explanation before giving consent.
   c. The risks, side effects, and benefits of treatment and other treatment options are explained.
   d. The parent(s) and child make treatment decisions in conjunction with the physician.

Chapter **1** **Introduction to Nursing Care of Children**

7. The nurse is presenting an in-service to a group of new graduate nurses about factors that influence learning at all ages. Which statement by one of the participants indicates a correct understanding of the teaching?
   a. "A family's previous experience with children does not influence their need for teaching."
   b. "A family's cultural beliefs will not interfere when teaching a family about care at home."
   c. "Children require teaching to be adapted to their developmental age rather than the chronologic age of the child."
   d. "Children require teaching to be conducted by a child life specialist for the child to best learn the material."

8. Which nursing interventions are for risk nursing diagnosis? *(Choose all that apply.)*
   a. Reduce the cause or related factors.
   b. Monitor for onset of problem.
   c. Support coping mechanisms.
   d. Eliminate risk factors.
   e. Prevent the problem.

2 Family-Centered Nursing Care

Review *Communicating with Children and Families* in Chapter 3 of your textbook.

STUDENT LEARNING EXERCISES

Definitions

Match each term with its definition.

1. _____ Coping

2. _____ Culture

3. _____ Discipline

4. _____ Ethnicity

5. _____ Ethnocentrism

6. _____ Nuclear family

a. The sum of the values, beliefs, and traditions of a particular ethnic or social group passed down from generation to generation

b. A family consisting of two generations, parents and children, who live together and are somewhat isolated from other close relatives

c. Condition of belonging to a particular group of people—either religious, racial, national, or cultural—who share a race, language, religion, traditions, values, food preferences, literature, or folklore

d. The structure a parent sets in a child's life

e. Efforts directed toward managing and solving various problems, events, and stressors

f. The opinion that the beliefs and customs of one's own ethnic group are superior to beliefs and customs of others

The Family and Nursing Care

7. How has family structure in the United States changed in the last 30 years?

_____

_____

8. Give three examples of a nontraditional family.

a. _____

b. _____

c. _____

Healthy versus Dysfunctional Families

9. To successfully resolve conflict, families need:

a. _____

b. _____

c. _____

Classify the following coping strategies as either internal (I) or external (E).

10. _____ Seeks support strategies

11. _____ Uses humor

12. _____ Relies on the family group

13. _____ Seeks spiritual support

14. _____ Maintains flexibility in family roles

Answer as either true (T) or false (F).

15. _____ Family conflict usually ends when the parents divorce.

16. _____ The rate of adolescent pregnancy has been rising since the 1990s.

17. _____ Infants of teenage mothers are at an increased risk for low birth weight and sudden infant death.

18. _____ Child abuse may be physical, sexual, or emotional, or it may take the form of neglect.

Cultural Influences in Pediatric Nursing

Answer as either true (T) or false (F).

19. _____ Culture plays a major role in influencing parenting practices.

20. _____ Mormons are not permitted to receive blood transfusions.

21. _____ In Asian culture, the elders in a family are usually highly respected.

22. _____ In Islamic culture, women gain status as they get older.

23. _____ In Japanese culture, prolonged eye contact is considered rude.

24. _____ Hispanics living in the United States are a homogeneous cultural group.

25. _____ Coining is a form of dermabrasion used as traditional treatment in some cultures.

Parenting

26. The three styles of parenting are:

    a. _____

    b. _____

    c. _____

Answer as either true (T) or false (F).

27. _____ Children with authoritarian parents tend to be self-confident.

28. _____ A parent with an authoritative parenting style would not be likely to discuss family rules with a child.

29. _____ Permissive parents seem to have little control over their child's behavior.

30. _____ A child with permissive parents is usually independent and respectful of others.

31. Describe characteristics of the three temperament categories developed by Chess and Thomas (1996).

Easy: _____

Difficult: _____

Slow-to-warm-up: _____

Discipline

32. The purpose of discipline is to:

_____

33. What are the three essential components of effective discipline?

a. _____

b. _____

c. _____

34. Describe the disciplinary technique of *redirection*.

_____

_____

_____

_____

35. How should a parent use *time out?*

_____

_____

36. List four problems associated with corporal punishment as a method of discipline.

a. _____

b. _____

c. _____

d. _____

37. What is behavior modification?

_____

_____

Answer as either true (T) or false (F).

38. _____ Reasoning is an effective method of discipline for toddlers and preschoolers.

39. _____ Reasoning is best accomplished with statements that begin with "You."

40. _____ Logical consequences are related directly to the child's misbehavior.

41. _____ Consistency is essential when parents are using a behavior modification program.

SUGGESTED LEARNING ACTIVITIES

1. Recall a client whose cultural background or religious beliefs were very different from yours. What were your initial feelings about caring for that client? Did you encounter any difficulties in establishing a therapeutic relationship with that client? How did you resolve them? Would you do anything differently if you cared for another client with a similar background or beliefs?

2. Interview members of a nontraditional family to learn about positive and negative aspects of their particular family structure.

STUDENT LEARNING APPLICATION

Enhance your learning by discussing your answers with other students.

Five-year-old Marcel has been admitted to the hospital for treatment of bacterial meningitis. Marcel had complained of a headache and sore neck for 2 days, so his grandmother gave him an herbal tea to relieve his discomfort. He was brought to the hospital by emergency personnel after he collapsed at home. Marcel and his 19-year-old mother, Keisha, live with his grandmother. Marcel's grandmother is his primary caretaker at home. However, his mother has been staying with him in the hospital since he was admitted.

When you enter the room, you notice Keisha standing by Marcel's crib. She seems to be praying softly. She says to you, "I am so afraid that Marcel is going to die." Later that day, another nurse, who overheard your conversation with Keisha makes the comment, "Can you believe this mom? She's worried about him dying and all she does is sit by his crib and pray. He wouldn't be so sick if she had brought him to the doctor instead of trying to treat the problem at home."

1. What type of family is described in this scenario?

2. Keisha explains that her family are Jehovah's Witnesses. How could the family's religious beliefs affect Marcel's treatment?

3. Identify a coping strategy Keisha used in this scenario.

4. What might you do or say in response to Keisha's comment, "I am so afraid that Marcel is going to die?"

5. How could you respond to the comments about Keisha made by the other nurse?

Choose the best answer.

1. During a home visit the nurse observes a father giving an explanation to a child who does not understand why he is being punished. Which parenting style is used in this situation?
   a. Autocratic
   b. Authoritarian
   c. Authoritative
   d. Permissive

2. Which are characteristics of a child whose parents use a permissive parenting style?
   a. Disobedient, disrespectful
   b. Inquisitive, assertive
   c. Insecure, shy
   d. Dependable, sensitive

3. A parent tells the nurse that she puts her 4-year-old in a time-out chair in the corner for 4 minutes when he misbehaves. The parent asks the nurse, "Am I doing time-out correctly?" How should the nurse respond?
   a. "Yes, you are using time-out correctly."
   b. "You should put the time-out chair in the center of activity."
   c. "I would increase the length of time-out to eight minutes."
   d. "Do you talk about the misbehavior while the child is in the chair?"

4. Which statement about corporal punishment is true?
   a. Spanking will effectively eliminate a specific misbehavior.
   b. Spanking is appropriate for the younger child who does not understand explanations.
   c. Spanking teaches the child that violence is an acceptable action.
   d. Spanking reinforces respect for parental authority.

5. Which example indicates that a parent understands the principles of behavior modification for a 7-year-old who dawdles and is argumentative about getting ready for school every morning?
   a. The child can go to the toy store after school if he or she gets dressed right away.
   b. The child gets a new book when he or she cooperates with getting dressed for 5 days.
   c. The child is reminded each morning that if he or she dawdles she will miss the bus.
   d. When the child dawdles, the parent tells the child the reward is canceled.

6. Which statement demonstrates an effective reasoning technique?
   a. "You are not being very nice when you throw toys at your friend."
   b. "I wouldn't throw that toy if I were you."
   c. "Your friend gets upset when you throw the toys at her. She thinks you don't like her."
   d. "I won't let you play at your friend's house if you throw toys."

7. An example of an external family coping strategy is:
   a. participating in self-help groups.
   b. using humor.
   c. reframing the meaning of a problem.
   d. joint problem solving among members.

8. Compulsory prayer five times a day is a religious practice in:
   a. Christian Science.
   b. Hinduism.
   c. Islam.
   d. Judaism.

9. The nurse is conducting a family assessment on a traditional family of six people, two parents, four children. Which aspect(s) of affective function (personality maintenance function) should the nurse consider during the assessment? *(Choose all that apply.)*
   a. Trust and nurturing
   b. Connectedness and separateness
   c. Provision and allocation of resources
   d. Prevention of medical and dental health practices
   e. Belonging and identity
   f. Guidance and transmission of cultural beliefs

10. The nurse is preparing a presentation on various practices of different religions. What information should the nurse include in the presentation?
    a. Roman Catholics do not permit organ donation.
    b. Hindus do not have specific rituals related to death.
    c. Jehovah's Witnesses may accept alternatives to blood transfusion.
    d. Mormons may refuse medical treatment.

3 Communicating with Children and Families

Review *Family-Centered Nursing Care* in Chapter 2 of your textbook.

HELPFUL HINT

Review *Family-Centered Nursing Care* in Chapter 2 of your textbook.

STUDENT LEARNING EXERCISES

Definitions

Match each term with its definition.

1. _____ Empathy

2. _____ Empowerment

3. _____ Active listening

4. _____ Therapeutic relationship

5. _____ Sensory information

6. _____ Self-esteem

a. Information gained from sight, taste, touch, smell, and hearing
b. The personal value that individuals place on themselves
c. Seeing a situation from another person's perspective while remaining objective
d. Balance between appropriate involvement and professional separation
e. Attending to another person to gain an understanding of the actual and the implied message
f. Actions taken to enable another person to participate fully in decision making

Components of Effective Communication

Answer as either true (T) or false (F).

7. _____ Cultural differences among people can hinder communication.

8. _____ Touch communicates more meaning for a younger child than for an older child.

9. _____ The child or family members may feel intimidated when the nurse stands over them while talking.

10. _____ A nurse watching a television program with the child is an example of communicating attentiveness to the child.

11. _____ Children will be more talkative and more apt to engage in conversation when asked close-ended questions.

12. _____ In some cultures, making eye contact is considered rude.

13. _____ Infants are too young to sense tone of voice.

14. _____ A nurse talking to a child with her hands on her hips is an example of a closed body posture.

15. _____ An appropriate time to teach a 4-year-old about surgery is immediately after the parents have gone home.

Family-Centered Communication

16. What is meant by the term *family-centered care?*

_____

17. List five key components of open communication in a family-centered care environment.

a. _____

b. _____

c. _____

d. _____

e. _____

18. How can the nurse establish rapport with families? _____

_____

_____

19. List seven strategies that may be useful in managing the conflicts that can arise with families.

a. _____

b. _____

c. _____

d. _____

e. _____

f. _____

g. _____

Transcultural Communication: Bridging the Gap

20. Why is it important for nurses to know about different cultures?

_____

_____

Therapeutic Relationships: Developing and Maintaining Trust

21. List three behaviors that indicate the nurse is overinvolved with a family or child.

a. _____

b. _____

c. _____

Nursing Care: Communicating with Children and Families

Answer as either true (T) or false (F).

22. _____ The optimal time to prepare a toddler for a painful procedure is just before the procedure is to be done.

23. _____ Showing children the treatment room before a procedure will heighten their anxiety.

24. _____ It is better not to tell children how long a painful procedure will take unless they ask.

25. _____ Once a procedure is completed, it is better to let the child forget about it.

Rewrite each of the following statements so that they are appropriate for addressing a 6-year-old child.

26. "It's time for your dressing change." _____

_____

27. "I am going to get you on the floor now." _____

_____

28. "I am going to give you a shot." _____

_____

29. "Let's get your vital signs." _____

_____

Communicating with Children with Special Needs

30. Suggest three strategies the nurse could use to communicate with a child with a severe visual impairment.

    a. _____

    b. _____

    c. _____

31. Suggest three strategies for communicating with a deaf child.

    a. _____

    b. _____

    c. _____

32. Suggest three strategies for communicating with a child with a profound neurologic impairment.

    a. _____

    b. _____

    c. _____

SUGGESTED LEARNING ACTIVITIES

1. Review Table 3-4 in your textbook. Think about the words you use when talking to children. How often have you used potentially ambiguous, hard to understand, or unfamiliar language? Make a conscious effort to use clear, softer, and more familiar language. Once you have had the opportunity to try this "new" language, consider its effects. What were the children's reactions to each style of communication?

STUDENT LEARNING APPLICATIONS

Enhance your learning by discussing your answers with other students.

A mother brings her 4-year-old son, Juan, to the pediatrician's office for a well-child examination. The physician completes the examination and reminds Juan's mother that he is due for immunizations during this visit. The nurse walks into the examination room holding a syringe in her hand. She looks at Juan and says, "This shot is so you won't get diphtheria, pertussis, or tetanus. I am going to put the needle in your leg (points to thigh area). You can cry or yell, but I need you to keep your leg still. It's going to hurt." She gives the injection and says, "Here is a band-aid to put on the sore spot. That wasn't too bad, was it?" The nurse leaves the room before Juan has a chance to respond.

1. What effective communication techniques were used by this nurse?

2. What communication pitfalls do you recognize in this nurse-child interaction?

3. What suggestions can you offer to make the nurse's communication more effective?

Martina is a 3-year-old girl who was diagnosed with liver failure. Martina is deaf. Her mother, who is present, speaks Spanish but understands some English. When Jan, the nursing student, enters Martina's room the child cries and wants to be held by her mother. Jan approaches Martina to take vital signs, but the child cries even louder.

1. What does Martina's behavior communicate to you?

2. What should Jan do about measuring vital signs at this time?

3. How can Jan establish rapport with Martina? With her mother?

4. What measures should Jan take to communicate with Martina? With her mother?

REVIEW QUESTIONS

Choose the best answer.

1. A 5-year-old is scheduled for a CT scan of her head. What is the best time for her mother to initiate a discussion about the procedure?
   a. Immediately before the procedure begins
   b. Two hours before the procedure
   c. The day before the procedure
   d. A few days before the procedure

2. Which action indicates the nurse understands the components of effective communication?
   a. The nurse stands right next to the chair, in which the child is seated.
   b. The nurse asks about hobbies in which the child is involved.
   c. The nurse speaks in a loud voice to a child with a hearing impairment.
   d. The nurse talks with her arms folded across her chest.

3. An adolescent tells the nurse, "I don't like this hospital room." Which response to the statement indicates active listening?
   a. "Don't you know this is the best room in the house?"
   b. "Let me see whether there are other rooms available."
   c. "What's wrong with this room?"
   d. "So, you would prefer a different room?"

4. The developmentally appropriate strategy to use when doing preoperative teaching for a 10-year-old is to:
   a. keep explanations under 5 minutes.
   b. organize information sequentially.
   c. use picture books about having an operation.
   d. speak in short, simple sentences.

5. A hearing impaired child needs a cast. What can the nurse do to facilitate communication with the child throughout the cast application process?
   a. Face the child when speaking to him or her.
   b. Speak at a slower pace than usual.
   c. Talk clearly and directly into the child's ear.
   d. Keep gestures to a minimum.

6. Which description is an example of a nurse with an open body posture?
   a. Speaking to a child with head bowed.
   b. Shifting weight from one leg to the other while speaking.
   c. Leaning away from the child while talking.
   d. Talking while hands are moving freely.

7. A child has just been diagnosed with type 1 diabetes mellitus. The child's father tells the nurse, "My wife will be back in the morning. Before she left, she told me that she has a lot of questions about what to do." What is the most appropriate response for the nurse to make at this time?
   a. "You will be meeting with the clinical specialist tomorrow. Ask her tomorrow."
   b. "Did the clinical specialist give you any papers to read? If not, I'll get a pamphlet for you."
   c. "Your wife might want to write down her questions so she won't forget anything when she comes back tomorrow."
   d. "Why don't you tell me what information you received from the clinical specialist today?"

8. The nurse is caring for a 5-year-old child after an appendectomy. Which communication approach would be acceptable for the nurse to use during a dressing change? *(Choose all that apply.)*
   a. Use simple, short sentences to explain the dressing change.
   b. Set a consequence if the child does not allow the dressing change to take place at the agreed time.
   c. Demonstrate on a doll what will take place during the dressing change.
   d. Tell the child that the dressing change will take place the following day.
   e. Allow the child to choose a popsicle to eat after the dressing change is complete.

Chapter **3** **Communicating with Children and Families**

4 Health Promotion for the Developing Child

HELPFUL HINT

Review growth and development in a developmental psychology textbook.

STUDENT LEARNING EXERCISES

Definitions

Match each term with its definition.

1. _____ Cephalocaudal

2. _____ Chronologic age

3. _____ Developmental age

4. _____ Growth spurts

5. _____ Heredity

6. _____ Learning

7. _____ Nutrients

8. _____ Proximodistal

a. Progression from midline to periphery
b. Age based on functional behavior
c. Transmission of genetic characteristics
d. Progression from head to toe
e. Behavior changes that occur as a result of maturation and experience with environment
f. Age in years
g. Brief periods of rapid increase in growth rate
h. Foods that supply the body with elements necessary for metabolism

Match each type of play with its description.

9. _____ Dramatic play

10. _____ Familiarization

11. _____ Symbolic play

a. Use of games and interactions that represent an issue or a concern
b. Use of materials associated with health care in creative, playful activities
c. Children act out roles and experiences that happened to them or someone else or that they fear

Overview of Growth and Development

Fill in the blanks.

12. Nurses need to have an understanding of growth and development to design care plans

that are _____.

13. An increase in physical size is referred to as _____.

14. Physical change in the complexity of body structures that enables higher-level functioning is

known as _____.

15. _____ is an increase in capabilities resulting from growth, maturation, and learning.

16. Changes in behavior that occur as the result of both maturation and experience with the environment are called _____.

17. Nurses must be familiar with normal patterns of growth and development so that _____ can be detected and treated early.

18. Next to each age write the corresponding stage of growth and development.

    a. 8 years _____

    b. 2 years _____

    c. 17 years _____

    d. 10 months _____

    e. 4 years _____

    f. 3 weeks _____

19. List three parameters used to measure growth in infants and children.

    a. _____

    b. _____

    c. _____

20. An infant's birth weight doubles by _____ and triples by _____.

21. _____ is an indicator of brain growth.

22. Primary dentition consists of _____ teeth; permanent teeth number _____.

Principles of Growth and Development

Match each pattern of growth and development with its example.

23. _____ Cephalocaudal

24. _____ General to specific

25. _____ Proximodistal

26. _____ Simple to complex

a. An infant responds to abdominal pain by flailing the extremities; the child responds by guarding the abdomen.
b. A toddler uses two-word sentences; a preschooler tells stories.
c. In the embryo, the trachea develops first, followed by outward development of the bronchial tree.
d. The infant can lift his or her head before being able to lift his or her trunk.

27. The first growth spurt occurs during _____; the second during _____.

28. Define *critical period*. _____

_____

_____

Chapter **4** **Health Promotion for the Developing Child**

Answer as either true (T) or false (F).

29. _____ Environmental factors influence growth and development prenatally and after birth.

30. _____ Standard growth curves are appropriate for assessing children regardless of racial or ethnic background.

31. _____ Children may regress to an earlier stage of development when they are stressed.

32. _____ Only inherited diseases affect growth and development.

33. _____ Parenting practices are dependent on the child's temperament.

Theories of Growth and Development

Match each stage of Piaget's theory with the example that is characteristic of that stage.

34. _____ Sensorimotor

35. _____ Preoperational

36. _____ Concrete operations

37. _____ Formal operations

a. Distinguishes fact from fantasy
b. Exhibits magical thinking
c. Develops sense of object permanence
d. Thinks abstractly

Identify which of Freud's stages of psychosexual development is represented by each of the following.

38. Child explores the world with the mouth: _____

39. Child initially demonstrates aggression toward the same-sex parent: _____

40. Child develops an adult view of sexuality: _____

41. Child learns to control the elimination processes: _____

42. Child typically prefers same-sex friends: _____

Fill in the blanks in the following statements to complete the developmental tasks of Erikson through adolescence.

43. Trust versus _____.

44. _____ versus shame and doubt.

45. _____ versus guilt.

46. Industry versus _____.

47. _____ versus role confusion.

Match each level of Kohlberg's theory with its example.

48. _____ Preconventional morality

49. _____ Conventional morality

50. _____ Postconventional morality

a. "I'll be good in school to make Daddy happy."
b. "I won't hit them because Mommy will yell at me."
c. "I won't blast my radio in the dorm. It is not fair to the other students."

Theories of Language Development

Fill in the blanks.

51. Language development closely parallels _____ development.

52. Receptive language is the ability to _____.

53. Expressive language is the ability to _____.

54. _____ is the infant's first method of communication.

Influences of Heredity on Growth and Development

55. What is heredity? _____

_____

56. List three interventions that nurses might use when working with families with genetic abnormalities.

a. _____

b. _____

c. _____

57. DNA is the basic building block of _____ and _____.

58. Genes may have two or more alternate forms called _____.

59. _____ are any of the 22 chromosome pairs that are not sex chromosomes.

60. A(n) _____ is a photograph of chromosomes arranged in pairs from largest to smallest.

Match each term with its description.

61. _____ Autosomal dominant disorder

62. _____ Autosomal recessive disorder

63. _____ Heterozygous

64. _____ Homozygous

65. _____ Monosomy

66. _____ Multifactorial disorder

67. _____ Polyploidy

68. _____ Teratogen

69. _____ Translocation

70. _____ Trisomy

71. _____ X-linked recessive disorder

a. Entire single chromosome is missing
b. Pair of alleles that are not identical
c. Carried on the X chromosome in females
d. Part or all of a chromosome is attached to another
e. An abnormal dominant gene is paired with a normal gene
f. An entire single chromosome is added
g. Pair of alleles is identical
h. Both alleles are abnormal
i. One or more sets of chromosomes is added
j. Results from interaction between genetic susceptibility and environmental factors during the prenatal period
k. Agent in the environment that causes birth defects

Assessment of Growth

72. Why are the child's height, weight, and head circumference plotted on standardized growth charts at every well-child checkup?

_____

_____

Assessment of Development

73. List four methods of assessing development.

a. _____

b. _____

c. _____

d. _____

74. The Denver Developmental Screening Test II (DDST-II) assesses development in which four functional areas?

a. _____

b. _____

c. _____

d. _____

Answer as either true (T) or false (F).

75. _____ When completing the DDST-II, the nurse should ask the parents whether the child behaved normally during the screening.

76. _____ The DDST-II is similar to an IQ test.

77. _____ Parents should be present during DDST-II screening.

78. _____ Nurses are able to diagnose developmental delays with the DDST-II.

The Nurse's Role in Promoting Optimal Growth and Development

79. What is *anticipatory guidance?* _____

_____

80. What are questions that the nurse should ask during the initial interview for a 4-year-old during a well-child check up?

_____

_____

_____

The Developmental Assessment

Fill in the blanks.

81. Define the term *play*. _____

_____

82. Practice play is also known as _____.

83. Symbolic play uses games and interactions to _____.

84. Games include _____.

Match each type of play with its description.

85. _____ Associative

86. _____ Cooperative

87. _____ Onlooker

88. _____ Parallel

89. _____ Solitary

a. Independent play
b. Child observing others playing
c. Organized play with group goals
d. Side-by-side play without interaction
e. Group play without group goals

Health Promotion

Answer as either true (T) or false (F).

90. _____ Immunizations are effective at decreasing childhood infectious diseases.

91. _____ Because all states require immunizations for children attending school, obtaining parental informed consent before immunization is not necessary.

92. _____ The preferred site for intramuscular injections for infants and toddlers is the deltoid muscle.

93. _____ Acetaminophen can be given to relieve the discomfort associated with vaccine administration.

94. _____ When administering more than one injection, the nurse should give the vaccines with separate syringes.

95. _____ An otherwise healthy child with a low-grade fever should not be immunized at this time.

Match each nutrient with its function.

96. _____ Carbohydrates

97. _____ Fats

98. _____ Proteins

99. _____ Water

100. _____ Vitamins/minerals

a. Builds and maintains body tissue
b. Transports nutrients to and waste away from cells
c. Major dietary source of energy
d. Regulates metabolic processes
e. Play a role in maintaining body temperature

101. Why is dietary fat intake not restricted in children younger than 2 years? _____

102. After age 3 years, fats should comprise no more than _____ % of daily calories.

103. Why is it important to gather data about a hospitalized child's food preferences?

_____

104. List three methods of obtaining a dietary history.

    a. _____

    b. _____

    c. _____

105. What is the leading cause of death in children? _____

SUGGESTED LEARNING ACTIVITIES

1. Observe pediatricians or nurse practitioners performing well-child assessments. How did they establish trust with the child and parents? How did they go about assessing the child's growth? How did they assess development? How did they convey their findings to the child's parents? Were they able to work effectively with both the child and the parents?

2. Chart the height, weight, and head circumference of at least three children (an infant, a young child, and a school-age child or adolescent) on a standardized growth chart. Write a brief interpretation of your findings.

STUDENT LEARNING APPLICATIONS

Enhance your learning by discussing your answers with other students.

The Savons brought 12-month-old Amy to the pediatrician for a well-baby checkup. They tell you they are concerned because Amy is not as tall as her brother was at 12 months and because she cannot walk yet. You plot her height, weight, and head circumference and find that these measurements fall within the same growth channel as on her previous visits. You have training in administering the DDST-II. You use this screening tool with Amy and find that she has no delays. Her immunizations are up to date. From a dietary history, you learn that she is drinking low-fat (2%) milk from a cup.

1. How would you interpret Amy's growth charts for the family?

2. Amy's parents express relief that she "passed the IQ test" when you interpret the results of the DDST-II for them. How would you respond to that?

3. What immunizations are needed at this time?

4. What anticipatory guidance would you give to the Savon family?

5. What concerns do you have about this situation?

6. How would you determine whether the parents' concerns about Amy's growth and development are alleviated?

Choose the best answer.

1. Which developmental stages are periods of rapid physical growth?
   a. Infancy and toddlerhood
   b. Infancy and adolescence
   c. Toddlerhood and preschool age
   d. Middle childhood and adolescence

2. Cephalocaudal development follows:
   a. the pattern of myelinization.
   b. the development of the bronchial tree.
   c. language development.
   d. neuromuscular development.

3. An infant responds to an injection by crying and flailing the extremities, whereas a preschooler responds by rubbing the injection site. This is an example of what pattern of development?
   a. cephalocaudal.
   b. proximodistal.
   c. general to specific.
   d. simple to complex.

4. A child's growth and development are affected by: *(Choose all that apply.)*
   a. Cultural background
   b. Heredity
   c. Socioeconomic status
   d. Immunizations
   e. Safety

5. Which theorist described how children learn?
   a. Erikson
   b. Freud
   c. Kohlberg
   d. Piaget

6. Teaching about safety to school-age children should be geared toward their:
   a. parents.
   b. chronologic age.
   c. cognitive level of development.
   d. ability to answer questions.

7. Parents of a preschooler are concerned because she wants "to marry" her father and told her mother to "go outside and get hit by a car." The nurse realizes that the:
   a. family should seek counseling.
   b. preschooler's behavior is normal.
   c. preschooler needs to be seen by a social worker.
   d. parents are not addressing the child's need for initiative.

8. The secondary dietary source of energy is:
   a. carbohydrates.
   b. fats.
   c. proteins.
   d. vitamins.

9. An adolescent who has been losing weight will record everything he eats for 3 days. This is an example of:
   a. an anthropometric measurement.
   b. cultural influences on diet.
   c. dietary guidelines.
   d. a dietary history.

25

10. Nurses can prevent childhood injuries by:
   a. modeling safety practices.
   b. educating parents through anticipatory guidance.
   c. supporting legislation that advocates safety measures.
   d. all of the above.

11. When children play board games, they learn that taking turns is rewarded and that cheating is not rewarded. This fosters their:
   a. physical development.
   b. cognitive development.
   c. emotional development.
   d. moral development.

12. Which pair of anthropometric data reflect an 18-month-old's current nutritional status?
   a. Head circumference and skinfold thickness
   b. Body mass index and height
   c. Weight and midarm circumference
   d. Dietary history and weight

13. A 12-month-old child's immunization record indicates that only one set of immunizations was given at 2 months. The nurse knows that:
   a. the entire series of immunizations must be repeated.
   b. the OPV vaccine should be given now.
   c. it is dangerous to re-administer the hepatitis B vaccine.
   d. the DTaP vaccine and not the dT vaccine should be given.

14. The nurse is caring for an infant girl with hemophilia. The nurse realizes that:
   a. both parents must be carriers.
   b. hemophilia is an autosomal dominant disorder.
   c. her mother is a carrier and her father has hemophilia.
   d. the infant has been misdiagnosed.

15. The nurse is teaching a 16-year-old girl about immunizations. Which statement made by the adolescent indicates an understanding of the teaching?
   a. "I should receive a second dose of the varicella vaccine when I am an adult."
   b. "When I receive the Td booster, I should expect to feel flu-like symptoms for 2 or 3 days afterwards."
   c. "I should receive a vaccine for smallpox before I leave for college."
   d. "When I receive the HPV immunization it will be given as three separate doses, with the second dose 4 weeks after the first, and the third dose 12 weeks after that."

16. Which is a characteristic of Erikson's theory of development? (Choose all that apply.)
   a. A 3-month-old infant develops trust through consistent care.
   b. A 22-month-old toddler develops autonomy through magical thinking.
   c. A 4-year-old child develops initiative by avoiding disapproval.
   d. A 12 year-old school-age child develops industry by mastering useful skills.
   e. A 15 year-old adolescent develops identity by gaining independence from parents.
   f. A 21-year-old adult develops generativity by developing a mutual relationship with another person.

17. Place in correct order the stages of Piaget's theory of development.
   a. Preoperational with magical thinking
   b. Concrete operations with logical thinking
   c. Sensorimotor with object permanence
   d. Formal operations with analysis of situations

5 Health Promotion for the Infant

HELPFUL HINT

Review infant development in a developmental psychology textbook.

STUDENT LEARNING EXERCISES

Definitions

Match each term with its definition.

1. _____ Asphyxiation

2. _____ Critical milestones

3. _____ Developmental milestones

4. _____ Egocentrism

5. _____ Mistrust

6. _____ Object permanence

7. _____ Parent-infant attachment

8. _____ Pincer Grasp

9. _____ Sensorimotor stage

10. _____ Stranger anxiety

11. _____ Trust

a. Benchmarks of development indicating that the child is developing normally
b. Complete absorption in self
c. Foundation on which a healthy personality is built
d. Use of the index finger and thumb to pick up objects
e. State of suffocation that severely compromises oxygen delivery
f. Realization that things continue to exist when out of sight
g. Distress felt when infant is separated from caregivers
h. Negative resolution of Erikson's first developmental task
i. Developmental milestones that, if not reached, necessitate a full developmental assessment
j. Period in which child uses senses and movement to understand and control the environment
k. Sense of connection between parent and infant

Growth and Development of the Infant

Next to each activity, write the age at which the behavior generally first appears.

Age Choices

1–2 months   3 months   4–5 months   6–7 months   8–9 months   10–12 months

12. Begins to follow simple commands _____

13. Crying becomes differentiated _____

14. Rolls from abdomen to back _____

15. Smiles in response to others _____

16. Birth weight doubles _____

17. Can stand alone _____

27

18. Begins to experience stranger anxiety _____

19. Is alert for 1.5 to 2 hours _____

20. Reflexes dominate behavior _____

21. Can breathe when nose is obstructed _____

22. Pincer grasp develops _____

23. Birth weight triples _____

24. Is an obligate nose breather _____

25. Has beginning sense of object permanence _____

Fill in the blanks.

26. Why are infants vulnerable to respiratory infections? _____
_____

27. During infancy the heart rate _____ while the blood pressure _____.

28. _____ transmits additional IgA protection to the infant.

29. At what age does the ability to digest and absorb fats reach adult levels? _____

30. Because infants' renal systems are immature, they are prone to _____
_____.

Match each substage of Piaget's sensorimotor stage with its description.

31. _____ Reflex activity

32. _____ Primary circular reactions

33. _____ Secondary circular reactions

34. _____ Coordination of secondary schemata

a. Actions become intentional.
b. Begins to develop a sense of object permanence.
c. Activities become less reflexive and more controlled.
d. Behavior is dominated by reflexes.

Answer as either true (T) or false (F).

35. _____ Depth perception is present at birth.

36. _____ Lack of eye muscle control at two months of age requires evaluation.

37. _____ All newborn infants should be screened for hearing problems.

38. _____ By 10 months, an infant should respond to his or her name.

39. _____ An infant's social smile is a communication tool.

40. _____ Vocalization is a reflexive activity.

41. _____ Infants' expressive language skills exceed their receptive language skills.

42. Briefly describe how an infant develops a sense of suspicion and mistrust.

_____

_____

43. How is the parent-infant attachment strengthened?

_____

_____

44. Why does separation anxiety begin at about six months of age?

_____

_____

Health Promotion for the Infant and Family

Fill in the blanks.

45. Transplacental immunity lasts approximately _____ months.

46. Infant formula lacks the _____ properties and easy _____ of breast milk.

47. Give three examples of mothers who should not breastfeed their infants. _____

_____.

48. Weaning is the transition from breastfeeding or bottle feeding to _____.

49. If juices are heated before drinking, the _____ is destroyed.

Answer as either true (T) or false (F).

50. _____ Infants typically have 12 teeth by their first birthday.

51. _____ Aspirin is the drug of choice for alleviating teething discomfort.

52. _____ Parents can use a tiny bit of toothpaste on a washcloth to clean their infant's teeth.

53. _____ Substituting a pacifier for a bed-time bottle may prevent bottle mouth caries.

54. _____ All infants require fluoride supplements to promote the development of healthy teeth.

55. List four suggestions that may help parents console their infants.

a. _____

b. _____

c. _____

d. _____

56. List four suggestions that may help parents reduce their infant's irritability.

a. _____

b. _____

c. _____

d. _____

Fill in the blanks.

57. Temperature settings on hot water heaters should be no higher than _____ F.

58. Gates at the top and bottom of stairs should be in place when the child starts to _____.

59. Foods that pose an asphyxiation risk include _____

_____

60. What does the American Academy of Pediatrics recommend for preventing sudden infant death?

_____

_____

SUGGESTED LEARNING ACTIVITIES

1. Design a safety booklet for parents of infants.

2. Perform a developmental assessment on an infant. Assess fine and gross motor skills, language patterns, and psychosocial interactions. Determine whether the infant is functioning at the expected level.

STUDENT LEARNING APPLICATIONS

Enhance your learning by discussing your answers with other students.

Jamal, an 8-month-old, is being hospitalized for 2 weeks to receive antibiotic therapy.

1. What can the nurse do to facilitate parent-infant attachment during this period?

2. How can the nurse deal with Jamal's stranger anxiety?

3. What can the hospital staff do to facilitate Jamal's development of trust?

REVIEW QUESTIONS

Choose the best answer.

1. According to Piaget, an infant who intentionally shakes a rattle to hear the sound is in what substage?
   a. Reflexive
   b. Primary circular reactions
   c. Secondary circular reactions
   d. Coordination of secondary schemata

30

2. An 11-month-old enjoys picking up Cheerios one by one with the thumb and index finger and throwing them on the floor. This is an example of:
   a. egocentrism.
   b. pincer grasp.
   c. oral activity.
   d. reflexive activity.

3. Infants should turn their eyes and head toward a sound coming from behind at:
   a. birth.
   b. age 4 months.
   c. age 6 months.
   d. age 10 months.

4. An infant will develop a sense of mistrust if he or she is:
   a. adopted.
   b. hospitalized after birth.
   c. consistently ignored.
   d. sent to day care before 2 months of age.

5. Parent-infant attachment:
   a. is critical for survival.
   b. is essential for normal development.
   c. involves the infant as an active participant in the process.
   d. all of the above.

6. The parents of a 3-month-old with colic explain that, because their child does not sleep through the night, they feel very frustrated. The nurse's first action is to:
   a. provide information about normal sleep-wake cycles in a 3-month-old infant.
   b. suggest that they practice relaxation techniques.
   c. assure them that they are not bad parents.
   d. demonstrate how to soothe the infant.

7. Which statement suggests that the parent needs more information about infant nutrition?
   a. "I'll change from formula to whole milk at 6 months."
   b. "I'll introduce iron-fortified rice cereals at about 5 months."
   c. "I'll add new foods one at a time."
   d. "I'll introduce drinking from a cup gradually."

8. Appropriate finger foods for an 11-month-old infant are:
   a. crackers.
   b. raisins.
   c. lollipops.
   d. popcorn.

9. Which statement about immunity and immunizations is true?
   a. Breastfed infants do not need immunizations until they are weaned.
   b. Infants are prone to infectious diseases because of immature immune systems.
   c. Transplacental immunity lasts through the first year of life.
   d. Immunizations offer the infant total protection against infectious diseases.

10. Which infant is at risk for development of lead toxicity?
    a. The 10-month-old whose father crafts stained glass
    b. The 8-month-old living in a newly built house
    c. The 9-month-old whose toys are all made in the United States
    d. The 6-month-old whose out-of-town cousin has lead toxicity

11. The nurse is teaching new parents about the care of their recently circumcised infant. Which statement made by the parents would indicate a correct understanding of the instruction?
    a. "I should contact the primary health care provider if my infant has not had a wet diaper for more than 6 hours."
    b. "I should attach the diaper securely to add pressure and help stop the bleeding."
    c. "I should remove the crusty yellow material that forms around the penis with an alcohol swab."
    d. "I should place a petroleum-based product on the Plastibell for the next 2 days."

12. Which condition is associated with a markedly elevated bilirubin level? *(Choose all that apply.)*
    a. Appearance of jaundice 3 days after birth
    b. Jaundice of the feet
    c. Serum bilirubin of 15 mg/dL
    d. Yellow color of the skin on a breastfed infant
    e. Circumoral cyanosis

13. The nurse is teaching a class on growth and development to a group of pregnant mothers. What information should the nurse include in the teaching? *(Choose all that apply.)*
    a. A 2-month-old is an obligate nose breather and holds an object momentarily.
    b. A 4-month-old may begin drooling and bring hands together at midline.
    c. A 6-month-old may slow in weight gain and sit unsupported.
    d. An 8-month-old generally has more regular patterns of bowel and bladder elimination and may reach for toys.
    e. A 10-month-old can stand alone and should have a complete pincer grasp.
    f. A 12-month-old should have tripled his or her birth weight and can feed himself or herself with a spoon.

14. The nurse is teaching a group of newly graduated nurses who will be working on a pediatric unit about nutrition for infants. Which statement made by one of the new nurses would indicate a need for additional instruction?
    a. "Once solid food had been introduced, the infant usually shows a decreased interest in breast- or bottle-feeding."
    b. "Calcium-fortified fruit juices should not be introduced until an infant is at least 6 months of age."
    c. "The American Academy of Pediatrics recommends breastfeeding infants for the first 6 months of life."
    d. "Introduction of solids is required with breastfed infants to ensure the proper amount of nutrients are ingested."

6 Health Promotion during Early Childhood

HELPFUL HINT

Review toddler and preschool development in a developmental psychology textbook.

STUDENT LEARNING EXERCISES

Definitions

Match each term with its definition.

1. _____ Associative play
2. _____ Autonomy
3. _____ Caries
4. _____ Cooperative play
5. _____ Dysfluency
6. _____ Irreversibility
7. _____ Negativism
8. _____ Parallel play
9. _____ Physiologic anorexia
10. _____ Regression
11. _____ Ritualism
12. _____ Symbolic play
13. _____ Symbolic thought
14. _____ Transductive reasoning

a. Return to a behavior characteristic of an earlier stage
b. Inability to understand a process in reverse
c. Reasoning from particular to particular
d. Ability to function independently
e. Playing alongside but not with others
f. Tooth decay
g. Ability to allow a mental image to represent something that is not present
h. Decreased appetite relative to decreased caloric need
i. Group play without goals
j. Need to maintain sameness
k. Disorders in the rhythm of speech in which child knows what to say but is unable to do so
l. Games that represent an issue to be addressed
m. Opposition or resistance to the direction of others
n. Organized play with group goals

Growth and Development during Early Childhood

Fill in the blanks.

15. During early childhood, the average weight gain is _____ pounds per year.

16. Children should reach half of their adult height by _____ years of age.

17. All 20 deciduous teeth should be present by _____ years of age.

For each of the following, write T if the behavior first occurs during toddlerhood or P if it first occurs during the preschool years.

18. _____ Learns to walk well

19. _____ May have imaginary friends

20. _____ Handedness clearly established

21. _____ Exhibits negativism as an expression of independence

22. _____ Object permanence firmly established

23. _____ Anterior fontanel closes

24. _____ Gender identity fully established

25. _____ May use aggressive speech to gain attention

26. _____ Is in the preconceptual substage of Piaget's preoperational stage

27. _____ Thinking characterized by centration and irreversibility

28. _____ Stranger anxiety reaches another peak

29. _____ Obeys rules out of self-interest

30. _____ Magic thinking is common

Match each characteristic of preoperational thinking with its example.

31. _____ Animism

32. _____ Centration

33. _____ Egocentrism

34. _____ Irreversibility

35. _____ Magical thought

a. Aaron believes the television watches him while he sleeps.
b. Beth took a toy truck apart and can't put it back together.
c. Carla's brother is in the hospital. She believes she made him sick because she didn't want to play with him.
d. Diego is unable to follow a two-step direction.
e. Elgin took the crayons Fred was using and can't understand why Fred is upset.

Health Promotion for the Toddler or Preschooler and Family

Answer as either true (T) or false (F).

36. _____ After 12 months of age, low-fat or nonfat milk may be given.

37. _____ An appropriate serving size for solid food for the young child is 1 tablespoon of solid food per year of age.

38. _____ It is appropriate to substitute juice for milk.

39. _____ A toddler who eats little solid food but drinks a quart of milk per day is meeting the RDA.

40. _____ Food jags cause physiologic anorexia.

41. When should a child first visit the dentist? _____

_____

42. Why are bedtime rituals important for young children? _____

_____

43. Explain the difference between nightmares and night terrors. _____

_____

44. A child learns self-control through _____ and _____.

45. List four discipline techniques appropriate for the preschooler.

   a. _____

   b. _____

   c. _____

   d. _____

46. How can parents prevent drownings? _____

47. Why are booster seats in the car recommended for preschoolers weighing more than 40 pounds?

_____

48. What should preschoolers be taught to do in the event that their clothes catch on fire?

_____

_____

49. What do parents need to know about firearm safety? _____

_____

_____

50. What is included in teaching children about sexual abuse? _____

_____

_____

51. Most children are physiologically ready for toilet training by 18 to 24 months. What is the rationale for postponing it until later?

_____

_____

52. List four strategies parents can use to decrease the frequency of temper tantrums.

a. _____

b. _____

c. _____

d. _____

53. How can parents deal with sibling rivalry when a new baby is brought into the household?

_____

_____

54. How can parents help a child who stutters? _____

_____

_____

SUGGESTED LEARNING ACTIVITY

Interview the parents of a toddler. Discover how they deal with the child's negativism. How did the parents handle toilet training? Was it difficult or easy? If the child has temper tantrums, how do the parents handle them? Ask the parents what information would have been helpful for them to know before their child entered the "terrible 2s."

STUDENT LEARNING APPLICATIONS

Enhance your learning by discussing your answers with other students.

A mother brought 4-year-old Jonathan into the clinic for a well-child checkup. After the physical examination, she seems uncomfortable and hesitant but eventually tells you that she has found her son masturbating. She finds this very distressing because of her religious beliefs. She says, "I can't believe my little boy picked up such a filthy habit." She tells you that she has punished Jonathan by not letting him play with the other children in their neighborhood.

1. What is your personal reaction to the mother's story?

2. If you have personal misgivings about her actions or reactions, what could you do to help yourself remain nonjudgmental?

3. How would you explain Jonathan's sexuality to his mother while acknowledging the importance of her religious beliefs?

4. How could you use Kohlberg's theory to help the mother understand Jonathan's ability to distinguish right from wrong?

REVIEW QUESTIONS

Choose the best answer.

1. Which of the following represents a burn hazard in a toddler's home?
   a. Pots are placed on the front burners of the stove.
   b. The fireplace is covered with a screen that attaches to the wall.
   c. Electrical outlets are covered with plastic socket protectors.
   d. The hot water temperature is set at 110° F.

2. The nurse is talking to a group of parents about safety measures for toddlers. Which statement made by a parent indicates the need for additional teaching?
   a. "We should put our child in the carseat, even if we only drive down the street."
   b. "We will not allow our child to play alone on the swing set in the enclosed backyard."
   c. "We should put our cleaning supplies on the shelves above the sink."
   d. "We will not leave our child in the bathtub alone, even if there are only a few inches of water in the bathtub."

3. During a well-child checkup, a father asks the nurse if his 3-year-old son, who weighs 33 pounds, can use the seat belt instead of the carseat. The nurse's best response is:
   a. "He's old enough to use a shoulder harness and lap belt."
   b. "He should continue to use the carseat."
   c. "It's time to switch to a booster seat."
   d. "He'll be safest in a rear-facing carseat."

4. Which type of conceptual thinking provides a toddler with a sense of security?
   a. Animism
   b. Egocentrism
   c. Negativism
   d. Ritualism

5. Toddlers have temper tantrums because they:
   a. have limited language ability.
   b. are not getting enough attention.
   c. are unable to distinguish right from wrong.
   d. have poor parent-child attachments.

6. During a well-child checkup, the nurse notices that a toddler's teeth are brownish and speckled white. The nurse suspects that the child:
   a. does not brush his or her teeth.
   b. goes to sleep with a bottle of milk.
   c. eats too much candy.
   d. ingests too much fluoride.

7. According to Erikson, preschoolers who are encouraged to try new things and be creative will develop a sense of:
   a. autonomy.
   b. initiative.
   c. industry.
   d. integrity.

8. A parent tells the nurse that she is worried because her preschooler has an imaginary friend. The nurse explains that:
   a. the parent should enroll in parenting classes.
   b. the child should go to day care at least 3 days a week.
   c. imaginary friends are not unusual during the preschool period.
   d. the child should see a child psychologist.

9. While 5-year-old Isaac is hospitalized for an appendectomy he tells the nurse that he is in the hospital because he was bad. The nurse should:
   a. suspect child abuse and report it to the authorities.
   b. question the parents about their discipline methods.
   c. explain to the child why he is in the hospital.
   d. ignore the comment.

Chapter **6** **Health Promotion during Early Childhood**

10. A hospitalized 5-year-old thinks that the IV pole is a tall, skinny monster that is going to tie him or her up. This is an example of:
    a. animism.
    b. centration.
    c. egocentrism.
    d. magical thinking.

11. Which indication suggests that a 27-month-old is ready to begin toilet training? *(Choose all that apply.)*
    a. The child is able to sit and squat.
    b. The child notices when the diaper is wet.
    c. The child can remove own clothing.
    d. The child has a difficult time staying dry during the night.
    e. The child relapses often for long periods of time.

12. The nurse is talking to a group of parents about discipline for children 4 to 5 years of age. Which statement made by one of the parents would indicate a correct understanding of the teaching?
    a. "I can explain right from wrong to my child with an understanding of the consequences."
    b. "I should offer my child many choices to ensure a desirable outcome."
    c. "I can practice time-in when my child plays quietly while I am making dinner."
    d. "I should put my child in the time-out chair for 30 minutes or longer if my child hits me."

13. Which are language and cognitive milestones for a 15- to 18-month-old? *(Choose all that apply.)*
    a. Understands cause and effect
    b. Understands simple directions
    c. Points to six body parts
    d. Points to familiar objects
    e. Uses holographic speech
    f. Uses egocentric language

7 Health Promotion for the School-Age Child

HELPFUL HINT

Review school-age child development in a developmental psychology textbook.

STUDENT LEARNING EXERCISES

Definitions

Match each term with its definition.

1. _____ Caries

2. _____ Conservation

3. _____ Malocclusion

4. _____ Menarche

5. _____ Self-care children

a. Misalignment of the teeth
b. Ability to understand that certain properties of objects remain the same despite changes in appearance
c. Children who care for themselves after school
d. Onset of menstruation
e. Tooth decay

Growth and Development of the School-Age Child

Answer as either true (T) or false (F).

6. _____ Throughout the school-age years, boys are consistently taller and heavier than girls.

7. _____ The onset of puberty is signaled by the preadolescent growth spurt.

8. _____ Tonsil enlargement in the school-age child is always an abnormal finding.

9. _____ All permanent teeth are in place by age 12 years.

10. _____ Menarche occurs later in females who are obese.

11. Why is active play important for school-age children? _____

_____

_____

12. Why are school-age children more prone to dehydration than adults? _____

_____

13. Reversibility allows school-age children in the concrete operational stage to anticipate the results of their

_____.

14. School-age children understand the principle of conservation of _____ before they understand conservation of _____.

15. Why is collecting baseball cards an appropriate activity for school-age children? _____

_____

_____

16. Why do middle ear infections occur less frequently in school-age children than in younger children?

_____

_____

17. How do school-age children develop a sense of industry? _____

_____

_____

18. How is the developmental task of industry related to self-esteem? _____

_____

_____

19. How does friendship change as the school-age child matures? _____

_____

_____

Fill in the blanks.

20. Briefly describe each of the stages of moral development according to Kohlberg.

    a. Preconventional, stage 2: _____

    b. Conventional, stage 3: _____

    c. Conventional, stage 4: _____

21. For parents' moral teaching to be effective, they must:

    a. _____ in accordance with their own values.

    b. be consistent in their _____ of what the child should do.

    c. be consistent in administering _____ and _____.

Health Promotion for the School-Age Child and Family

22. Dietary recommendations for school-age children include:

    a. _____ ounces of grains

    b. _____ cups of vegetables

    c. _____ cups of fruits

    d. _____ ounces of protein

    e. _____ cups of dairy products

23. A 6-year-old needs about _____ hours of sleep, whereas a 12-year-old needs _____ hours.

24. How can parents foster a sense of responsibility in their children?

    _____

    _____

25. List three strategies parents can use to help their child succeed in school.

    a. _____

    b. _____

    c. _____

26. How can nurses act as advocates for self-care children?

    _____

    _____

27. What is the difference between school phobia and separation anxiety? _____

    _____

    _____

SUGGESTED LEARNING ACTIVITIES

1. Interview an elementary school teacher. Ask about the common stressors encountered by students in the teacher's class. How does the teacher's perception of student stressors compare with those identified in your textbook? What information does the teacher think school-age children need to help them cope more effectively with stress?

2. Choose one of the topics under "Sources of Stress in Children" in your textbook. Design a teaching plan focused on this topic and intended for a group of 8- to 10-year-old children. What makes this topic stressful? How can children in this age group cope with that stressor?

41

STUDENT LEARNING APPLICATIONS

Enhance your learning by discussing your answers with other students.

During a well-child checkup, the parents of 11-year-old Erica express their concern that their daughter seems to be heavier than "other children in her class, even the boys." After plotting Erica's height and weight on her growth chart, you find that her BMI is at the 90th percentile.

1. How would you collect information about Erica's eating habits? About her activity level?

2. How will you encourage Erica to participate in planning a weight reduction program for herself?

3. How will you encourage Erica to increase her activity level?

4. What guidance would you give Erica's parents about managing this problem?

REVIEW QUESTIONS

Choose the best answer.

1. The preadolescent growth spurt occurs:
   a. earlier in boys than in girls.
   b. earlier in girls than in boys.
   c. at about the same time in boys and girls.

2. Sex education for the 9-year-old should include information about:
   a. anatomy and physiology.
   b. body functions.
   c. what to expect during puberty.
   d. all of the above.

3. The nurse is teaching a group of school-age children about increased risks for having dental caries. Which statement made by one of the children would indicate a need for additional teaching?
   a. "I am at risk for dental caries because I wear braces."
   b. "I wear a mouth protector when I play sports to protect my teeth."
   c. "I had a cleft palate when I was young so I am at risk for dental caries."
   d. "I eat chocolate as a snack, which is better for my teeth."

4. Children in the intuitive thought stage:
   a. continue to exhibit egocentrism.
   b. are able to reverse their thinking.
   c. can classify objects into categories.
   d. decenter.

5. An appropriate coach for a child's basketball team:
   a. has a win-at-all-costs philosophy.
   b. is courteous to children, referees, and other coaches.
   c. divides the children into teams on the basis of age.
   d. all of the above.

6. An example of an activity that develops fine motor skills in the school-age child is:
   a. rollerblading.
   b. playing the guitar.
   c. playing chess.
   d. swimming.

7. The nurse is caring for a 9-year-old. The nurse should understand that the child is in the concrete operational stage and would exhibit which characteristic(s)? *(Choose all that apply.)*
   a. Egocentric thinking
   b. Understands historical time
   c. Ability to classify objects
   d. Doesn't understand another person's point of view
   e. Understands the rules but not the reason
   f. Doesn't make the distinction between accidental and intentional wrongdoing

8. *Healthy People 2020* objectives for school-age children include:
   a. increasing the proportion of children with disabilities who are older than 5 years of age to spend at least 40% of their time in regular education programs.
   b. increasing the proportion of children 2 through 16 years of age who play video games to less than 50%.
   c. increasing the proportion of children older than 2 years of age who consume at least 30% of their calories from fat.
   d. increasing the proportion of children 6 to 9 years of age who receive dental sealants on their molar teeth.

9. A child who fails to complete the developmental task of industry develops a sense of:
   a. shame and doubt.
   b. guilt.
   c. inferiority.
   d. confusion.

10. The nurse is talking about managing obesity with the parent of a 10-year-old child who has a BMI in the 85th percentile. Which statement made by the parent would indicate a correct understanding of the teaching?
    a. "I can use food as a reward if my child loses weight."
    b. "I should establish consistent times for meals and snacks."
    c. "I can keep unhealthy snacks in the house and give them to my child once a day."
    d. "I should allow my child to play video games after school and then exercise for 15 minutes."

11. Which personal/social skill would be noted in a 7-year-old child? *(Choose all that apply.)*
    a. Outgoing and boisterous
    b. Responsible and dependable
    c. Able to control anger and outbursts
    d. Has a sense of humor and tells jokes
    e. Has a strong sense of fairness and justice
    f. Develops clubs with secret codes and rituals

Chapter **7** **Health Promotion for the School-Age Child**

8 Health Promotion for the Adolescent

HELPFUL HINT

Review adolescent development in a developmental psychology textbook.

STUDENT LEARNING EXERCISES

Definitions

Match each term with its definition.

1. _____ Adolescence

2. _____ Autonomy

3. _____ Egocentrism

4. _____ Identity formation

5. _____ Primary sexual characteristics

6. _____ Puberty

7. _____ Pubescence

8. _____ Reproductive maturity

9. _____ Risk-taking behavior

10. _____ Secondary sex characteristics

11. _____ Sexual maturity rating (SMR)

a. Spermatogenesis in males and menstruation in females
b. Acquisition of psychosocial, sexual, and vocational identity
c. Period before sexual maturity
d. Capacity to be self-governing
e. Transition from childhood to adulthood
f. Internal and external reproductive organs
g. Stages of sexual maturation
h. Behavior that predisposes a person to harm
i. Concern with self
j. Achievement of reproductive maturity
k. Physical characteristics of males and females that have no direct role in reproduction

Adolescent Growth and Development

Fill in the blanks.

12. Physical maturation in girls occurs with the onset and establishment of _____.

13. Another term for the adolescent growth spurt is _____.

14. In girls, the appearance of _____ is the first sign of ovarian functioning.

15. Breast enlargement in boys is called _____.

16. An adolescent's chronologic age provides less information about physical development

    than does _____.

17. In boys, the first sign of pubertal changes is _____ .

18. The secretion of sex hormones (_____ in girls and _____ in boys) stimulates the development of breast tissue, pubic hair, and genitalia.

19. List five strategies for communicating effectively with teens.

a. _____

b. _____

c. _____

d. _____

e. _____

20. In adolescent development, what is meant by the term *"moratorium"?* _____

_____

_____

21. What functions do adolescent peer groups serve? _____

_____

_____

For questions 22 through 29, identify the period of adolescence (early, middle, late) during which the described behavior is most likely to occur.

22. Best friends are of the same sex. _____

23. Children react to an imaginary audience. _____

24. Emancipation from parents is common. _____

25. Children over-identify with glamorous role models. _____

26. Conflicts with parents escalate. _____

27. Conformity becomes less important. _____

28. Gang membership brings security. _____

29. This is the most frustrating time for parents. _____

Health Promotion for the Adolescent and Family

Answer as either true (T) or false (F).

30. _____ Lack of self-esteem and peer pressure play a role in determining a teen's sexual behavior.

31. _____ Adolescents require fewer calories during the period of peak height velocity (PHV).

32. _____ An avulsed tooth should be placed in a container of milk for transport.

33. _____ Because of peak height velocity (PHV), adolescents require at least 10 hours of sleep per night.

34. _____ Regular exercise promotes healthy sleep patterns.

35. _____ More teens die from injuries than from all other causes of death combined.

36. _____ Adolescents with tattoos may be injured during magnetic resonance imaging (MRI) scans.

Fill in the blanks.

37. In 2006, the CDC found that _____% of 9th through 12th graders had engaged in sexual activity.

SUGGESTED LEARNING ACTIVITY

Visit a teen pregnancy center in your community. Find out what services are offered, how teens are selected for the program, how the program is evaluated, and how it is funded. What other health promotion activities does the program provide for teens? Report your findings to your class.

STUDENT LEARNING APPLICATIONS

Enhance your learning by discussing your answers with other students.

You are invited to address a high school parent-teacher meeting to talk about early adolescent health.

1. What physical health information would you include? Why?

2. What developmental information would you include? Why?

3. What psychological health information would you include? Why?

REVIEW QUESTIONS

Choose the best answer.

1. According to Piaget, most adolescents achieve which stage?
   a. Sensorimotor
   b. Preoperational
   c. Concrete operations
   d. Formal operations

2. The adolescent growth spurt:
   a. occurs about 1 year after thelarche in girls.
   b. occurs 1 year before the onset of puberty.
   c. corresponds with spermatogenesis in boys.
   d. occurs later in girls than in boys.

3. In adolescence, sexual activity is usually related to:
   a. risk taking.
   b. alcohol or substance abuse.
   c. low self-esteem.
   d. all of these.

4. According to Erikson, a person who has not successfully completed the developmental task of adolescence will experience:
   a. shame and doubt.
   b. identity.
   c. role confusion.
   d. guilt.

5. Which of the following tools are used to assess sexual maturity?
   a. DDST-II
   b. Dubowitz
   c. Tanner
   d. Elkind

6. Which are *Healthy People 2020* objectives for adolescents? *(Choose all that apply.)*
   a. Increase the number of adolescents who graduate with a regular diploma 4 years after entrance into 9th grade.
   b. Reduce bullying and physical fighting among adolescents.
   c. Reduce pregnancies among adolescents.
   d. Increase the number of blood lead level tests given to adolescents after entrance into 10th grade.
   e. Improve access to resources for 13- to 18-year-old adolescents with mental illness.

7. In boys, peak height velocity (PHV) occurs during Tanner stages:
   a. 1 and 2.
   b. 2 and 3.
   c. 3 and 4.
   d. 4 and 5.

8. The nurse is teaching a 13-year-old with gynecomastia. What information should the nurse include about gynecomastia?
   a. "This condition is always bilateral and requires surgery."
   b. "This condition occurs in about 2/3 of adolescent males."
   c. "This condition usually occurs in late adolescence so other tests will be conducted."
   d. "This condition is seen in both girls and boys at this age."

9. The nurse addressing a group of adolescents discusses specific topics related to the adolescent period. Which statement made by one of the adolescents would indicate a need for additional teaching?
   a. "If I get my tongue pierced, I should watch for signs of an allergy to metal."
   b. "I could get a tattoo now and have it easily removed when I am an adult."
   c. "If I want to look tan I should use an over-the-counter lotion."
   d. "I should discuss birth control with my partner so that we are both responsible."

10. Which are characteristic(s) of middle adolescence? *(Choose all that apply.)*
    a. Shy and self-conscious
    b. Introspective and narcissistic
    c. Conflicts with parents increase
    d. Parental approval remains strong
    e. Extreme interest in the opposite sex occurs
    f. Expectations are more realistic and less self-serving

9 Physical Assessment of Children

HELPFUL HINT

Review the physical assessment of the infant and child in a nursing health assessment textbook.

STUDENT LEARNING EXERCISES

Definitions

Match each term with its definition.

1. _____ Auscultation

2. _____ Circumduction

3. _____ Crepitation

4. _____ Development

5. _____ Fasciculation

6. _____ Fremitus

7. _____ Growth

8. _____ History

9. _____ Inspection

10. _____ Obtund

11. _____ Palpation

12. _____ Percussion

13. _____ Systematic assessment

a. Vibration perceptible on palpation or auscultation
b. Organized method of collecting data
c. Use of touch to determine temperature, moisture, and organ placement
d. Circular movement of a limb or eye
e. Aggregate of subjective data that describe past and present health status
f. Tapping of the body to determine density, location, and size of organs
g. Evaluation of sounds produced by body
h. Observation to identify physical findings
i. Dry, crackling sound or sensation
j. Small, local, involuntary muscle contraction visible under the skin
k. To render dull or blunt
l. Change that occurs over time in functional, psychosocial, and cognitive behavior
m. Measurable physical and physiologic changes that occur over time

General Approaches to Physical Assessment

Answer as either true (T) or false (F).

14. _____ It is appropriate to auscultate the heart, lungs, and abdomen while an infant is sleeping.

15. _____ Stranger anxiety makes the physical examination of an older infant more difficult.

16. _____ Parents should not be present during a young child's physical examination.

17. _____ In all age groups, invasive procedures should be saved until the end of the examination.

18. _____ Adolescents should be allowed to participate in deciding who will be present during the physical examination.

19. _____ For adolescents, the physical examination proceeds from head to toe.

48

Techniques for Physical Examination

Fill in the blanks.

20. Using an ophthalmoscope is an example of _____ inspection.

21. In palpating the lymph nodes for general assessment, the nurse uses the _____.

22. In palpating the lymph nodes specifically for heat, the nurse uses the _____.

23. When percussing the liver, the nurse would expect to hear _____ sounds.

24. The _____ of the stethoscope is most effective in auscultating low-pitched sounds.

Match each type of history with its description.

25. _____ Complete history

26. _____ Episodic history

27. _____ Well-interim history

a. Information about a specific problem is added to an existing database
b. Information about a child from conception to present
c. Information gathered from last visit to current visit

Answer as either true (T) or false (F).

28. _____ Axillary temperatures are preferable to rectal temperatures because they are less invasive.

29. _____ The apical pulse is palpated to determine the position of the heart.

30. _____ All irregular heart rhythms in children require immediate attention.

31. _____ The respiratory rate in infants can be counted by observing the movement of the abdomen.

32. _____ An adolescent with a blood pressure of 130/80 mm Hg is considered prehypertensive.

33. Describe two ways of measuring the length of an infant. _____

_____

_____

34. Why is the head circumference measured at every visit until the child is three years old?

_____

_____

Fill in the blanks.

35. All scales must be _____ before use.

36. Chest circumference is measured at the _____.

37. Midarm circumference is a measure of _____ and _____.

38. An adolescent who is 5 feet, 2 inches tall and weighs 120.5 pounds has a body mass index (BMI) of _____.

39. To complete a growth chart on a child's height, the nurse should do the following:

    a. Use a chart appropriate for the child's _____ and _____.

    b. Find the child's age on the _____ axis.

    c. Find the child's height on the _____ axis.

    d. Mark where the two lines _____.

    e. Note the _____.

40. Depigmentation of the skin is called _____.

41. On a child, the nurse assesses skin turgor on the _____ or _____.

42. Unusual hair loss is called _____; excessive hair growth is called

_____.

43. When a child has head lice, nits are found in the _____.

44. Capillary refill should be within _____ seconds.

45. When assessing a child's face, the nurse examines cranial nerves _____ and _____.

46. Frequent wiping of the nose indicates that the child probably has _____.

47. The philtrum is the _____.

48. How does the nurse examine cranial nerve XII? _____

_____

49. By eliciting the gag reflex, the nurse assesses cranial nerve _____.

Match each test with its description.

50. _____ Sweep

51. _____ Hirschberg

52. _____ Ishihara

53. _____ Rinne

54. _____ Snellen

55. _____ Whisper

    a. Tests ability to hear by bone and air conduction
    b. Audiometric test for hearing loss
    c. Tests hearing acuity in an 8-year-old
    d. Tests color vision
    e. Tests corneal light reflex
    f. Tests visual acuity in a 12-year-old

Answer as either true (T) or false (F).

56. _____ Breathing tends to be more diaphragmatic in a school-age child than in a toddler.

57. _____ Before auscultating breath sounds, the nurse should have a toddler sit on the parent's lap.

58. _____ Normal breath sounds are called adventitious.

59. _____ The apical pulse is also identified as the point of maximal impulse (PMI).

60. _____ Auscultation of the heart is best done by listening with the bell of the stethoscope only.

61. _____ A pause between the closing of the pulmonic and aortic valves is a normal finding in children.

62. _____ Functional heart murmurs require immediate intervention.

63. When should adolescent females start performing monthly breast self-examinations?

_____

64. When assessing the abdomen, why does auscultation follow inspection? _____

_____

65. Describe how to test for rebound tenderness. _____

_____

_____

66. How can the nurse decrease adolescent anxiety during a genital examination? _____

_____

67. Why are adolescent males taught to do monthly testicular examinations? _____

_____

Answer as either true (T) or false (F).

68. _____ To test neurologic function in a child younger than 5 years of age, use the DDST-II.

69. _____ The nurse should test all the cranial nerves at the beginning of the physical examination.

70. _____ Obtunded is a term used to describe one of the altered levels of consciousness.

71. _____ As part of the neurologic examination, it is important to assess a toddler's orientation to person, place, and time.

72. _____ Depression may alter a child's ability to solve problems.

73. _____ Tests designed to assess cerebellar function vary with the child's age and development.

74. _____ Assessing a child's ability to balance evaluates cerebellar function.

75. _____ Responses to eliciting the Babinski reflex depend on the child's ability to walk.

76. _____ Neurologic "soft" signs are normal variants and require no further assessment.

STUDENT LEARNING ACTIVITIES

1. Perform a complete history and physical assessment on an infant, child, or adolescent. Describe your findings clearly and coherently in writing.

2. Complete the following chart, which reviews the physical examination of the various body systems and the developmental considerations for each aspect of the physical examination.

REVIEW OF PHYSICAL EXAMINATION

Area to be Assessed	What to Assess	Developmental Considerations
General appearance		
Head		
Hair		
Face		
Eyes		
Nose and sinuses		
Mouth		
Throat		
Neck		
Lungs		
Heart		
Breasts		
Abdomen		
Kidneys and bladder		
Bowels, rectum, and anus		
Genitalia		
Musculoskeletal system		
Neurologic system		

Enhance your learning by discussing your answers with other students.

During the physical assessment of an infant, child, or adolescent, many variables can alter either the process or the findings. Describe how you would handle a physical assessment in each of the following situations.

1. A toddler's parents are not present during the examination.

2. A school-age child's level of cognitive functioning is far below average.

3. An adolescent has moderately severe abdominal pain.

4. A 9-month-old is exhibiting a high degree of stranger anxiety.

5. A preschooler believes that undergoing the physical examination is punishment for being bad.

REVIEW QUESTIONS

Choose the best answer.

1. A 1-year-old child is at the pediatrician's office for a well-interim visit. When interviewing the parents, the nurse should:
   a. obtain a complete history from conception to the present.
   b. record information about the child's chief complaint.
   c. obtain a family history.
   d. gather data about what has occurred since the last visit.

2. Before auscultating a toddler's lungs, the nurse should:
   a. examine the child's ears and throat.
   b. ask the parent(s) to leave the room.
   c. allow the child to examine the stethoscope.
   d. do none of the above.

3. The nurse begins auscultation of the abdomen in the:
   a. RUQ.
   b. RLQ.
   c. LUQ.
   d. LLQ.

4. Which is an abnormal finding?
   a. Posterior fontanel is flat and soft in an 8-month-old infant.
   b. A 7-month-old sits by using hands for support.
   c. The isthmus of the thyroid gland is palpable in a 12-month-old child.
   d. A 5-year-old's pupils dilate when focusing on a distant object.

5. Which is a normal finding in a school-age child?
   a. Bone conduction is greater than air conduction.
   b. Cerumen is found in the external auditory meatus.
   c. Discharge is present in the ear canal.
   d. The tympanic membrane is stationary.

6. An assessment technique of the chest and lungs normally reserved for the advanced nursing practitioner is:
   a. inspection.
   b. auscultation.
   c. palpation.
   d. percussion.

7. The point of maximal impulse (PMI) is located at the fifth intercostal space in the midclavicular line after about age:
   a. 2 months.
   b. 18 months.
   c. 4 years.
   d. 7 years.

8. An example of a "soft" neurologic sign is:
   a. a short attention span.
   b. left handedness.
   c. nonmirroring movement of the extremities.
   d. none of the above.

9. Which sound occurs when parts of the lungs lose their lubricating fluid?
   a. High-pitched wheezing
   b. Pleural friction rub
   c. Rales
   d. Sonorous rhonchi

10. Which reflex is elicited by suddenly and briskly dorsiflexing the child's foot and applying moderate pressure?
    a. Achilles
    b. Babinski
    c. Clonus
    d. Patellar

11. Place in the correct order the sequence of assessments during an abdominal examination of a 4-year-old child.
    a. Palpation
    b. Auscultation
    c. Inspection
    d. Percussion

12. Place in the correct order the progression of walking for a child.
    a. Sits from standing position
    b. Maintains balance
    c. Steps with arms flexed
    d. Walks with support

13. Which characteristics are a neurologic "soft" sign? *(Choose all that apply.)*
    a. Adequate attention span
    b. Motor overflow
    c. Even perceptual development
    d. Dyslexia
    e. Hyperkinesis
    f. Clumsiness

14. The nurse is talking to a parent of a 12-year-old. Which statement made by the parent would indicate a need for follow-up?
    a. "I have noticed that my child has only grown 2 inches since the last physical examination."
    b. "My child has asked to wear corrective lenses instead of glasses."
    c. "I have noticed that the hem is always frayed on one side of my child's pants."
    d. "My child has had an extra heart sound since she was an infant."

10 Emergency Care of the Child

HELPFUL HINT

Review the anatomy and physiology of the cardiac and respiratory systems in the textbook.

STUDENT LEARNING EXERCISES

Definitions

Match each term with its definition.

1. _____ Cardiopulmonary resuscitation

2. _____ Extracorporeal membrane oxygenation

3. _____ Envenomation

4. _____ Hypothermia

5. _____ Ingestion

6. _____ Submersion injury

7. _____ Trauma

8. _____ ABCDEs

a. Injury from an external cause
b. Protocol performed when an individual's respiratory and cardiovascular systems require support to maintain vital functions
c. Cooling of body temperature to subnormal levels
d. Temporary method of providing cardiovascular, pulmonary, and circulatory support when other treatment is not effective
e. Swallowing of a potentially toxic substance
f. Critical components of the primary assessment of a critically ill or injured child: airway, breathing, circulation, disability, and exposure
g. Injuries resulting from a near-drowning incident
h. Injection of venom by an animal

General Guidelines for Emergency Nursing Care

9. List five interventions that can facilitate a more positive and comfortable emergency experience for a child and family.

   a. _____

   b. _____

   c. _____

   d. _____

   e. _____

10. List three strategies that the nurse can use when dealing with family members who are emotionally distressed after being told that their child's injuries are life threatening.

   a. _____

   b. _____

   c. _____

Match each medication with its use in pediatric emergency care.

11. _____ Activated charcoal

12. _____ Atropine sulfate

13. _____ Dextrose

14. _____ Epinephrine

15. _____ Naloxone

16. _____ Sodium bicarbonate

a. Reverses the effects of some narcotics
b. Treats symptomatic bradycardia
c. Treats bradycardia or asystolic arrest
d. Treats severe acidosis
e. Reduces drug absorption in toxic ingestions
f. Treats hypoglycemia

Growth and Development Issues in Emergency Care

Match each age group with the appropriate nursing interventions.

17. _____ Infant

18. _____ Toddler

19. _____ Preschooler

20. _____ School-age

21. _____ Adolescent

a. Ascertain child's level of understanding and allow time for questions.
b. Allow the child to have familiar objects to help him or her feel safe.
c. Use a soothing voice and touch, rock, or cuddle the child.
d. Explain procedures in detail; encourage choices.
e. Talk to the child throughout the procedure and explain how he or she can help.

The Family of a Child in Emergency Care

22. The two most common emotions felt by parents of children who are being cared for in an emergency setting are

_____ and _____.

23. The underlying cause of the anger that some parents express toward health care providers in an emergency setting is often the fear _____.

Emergency Assessment of Infants and Children

24. Describe the role of the triage nurse. _____

_____

_____

_____

25. A triage nurse performs an initial observation in an emergency setting, focusing on which three factors?

a. _____

b. _____

c. _____

26. List the components of the *primary assessment.*

A: _____

B: _____

C: _____

D: _____

E: _____

Answer as either true (T) or false (F).

27. _____ Respiratory rate of more than 60 breaths per minute is considered abnormal for a child of any age.

28. _____ Tachycardia and decreased peripheral perfusion are early signs of cardiovascular compromise in a child.

29. _____ Infants and young children have a higher percentage of fluid located in the intracellular compartment.

30. _____ For the first several months of life the presence of nasal secretions can cause respiratory compromise in infants.

31. _____ Nasal flaring on inspiration is an indicator of respiratory distress in infants and young children.

32. What are the four components of the *secondary assessment*?

F: _____

G: _____

H: _____

I: _____

33. What is the suggested order for measuring vital signs in children?

_____

_____

34. Identify the elements of a SAMPLE history.

S: _____

A: _____

M: _____

P: _____

L: _____

E: _____

35. Which laboratory tests are considered standard protocol in an emergency setting?

_____

36. Why is determining the child's weight essential in emergency care?

_____

Cardiopulmonary Resuscitation of the Child

37. What are the two most common causes of cardiopulmonary arrest in children?

    a. _____

    b. _____

38. Ventilations should be given at a rate of _____, or approximately

    one breath every _____ seconds.

39. What is the emergency intervention for an obstructed airway in a conscious child?

_____

40. What is the emergency intervention for an obstructed airway in an unconscious child?

_____

41. What is the rationale for NOT performing blind finger sweeps on infants and children?

_____

42. What is the emergency intervention for removal of a foreign object from an infant?

_____

43. Before and during cardiac compressions, the nurse feels for a pulse in the infant at the

    _____ ; for a child older than 1 year of age, at the

    _____.

44. According to the American Heart Association, chest compressions are performed at a rate of _____.

45. In the community setting, an automatic external defibrillator (AED) should be used on a child who has cardiac

    arrest after _____ cycles of CPR have been performed.

The Child in Shock

Indicate whether each statement refers to hypovolemic (H), cardiogenic (C), or distributive (D) shock.

46. _____ The most common type of shock seen in children

47. _____ Occurs when myocardial function is unable to produce cardiac output that meets the metabolic demands of the body

48. _____ Occurs when bacterial toxins are in the bloodstream

49. _____ Early signs include warm extremities and tachycardia

50. _____ Diuretics are prescribed because of increased intravascular volume

51. _____ Periorbital edema, crackles, and diaphoresis are clinical manifestations

52. _____ Initial treatment involves administration of colloids

Answer as either true (T) or false (F).

53. _____ Hypotension is an early sign of shock in children.

54. _____ An important assessment in hypovolemic shock is the child's neurologic status.

55. _____ Early signs of cardiogenic shock include hyperthermia or hypothermia.

56. _____ Enalaprilat, dopamine, and milrinone are the initial drugs of choice for treating distributive shock.

Pediatric Trauma

Answer as either true (T) or false (F).

57. _____ Injury is the leading cause of death in children.

58. _____ Injuries from blunt trauma are often less obvious, although more serious than injuries from penetrating trauma.

59. _____ Unrestrained individuals involved in an automobile accident are more likely to be injured than are restrained individuals.

60. _____ The largest number of pedestrian injuries occurs in children ages 5 to 9 years.

61. _____ An example of a penetrating injury is a gunshot wound.

62. State the goal of the *primary survey* in pediatric trauma._____

_____

63. Identify the four elements of the *primary survey* used in the management of pediatric trauma.

A. _____

B. _____

C. _____

D. _____

64. What is included in the *secondary survey?* _____

_____

65. Write two questions that the nurse should ask when obtaining a history for each type of injury.

Motor vehicle: ._____

_____

Fall: _____

_____

Penetrating injury: _____

_____

66. List five indicators of or physical findings that indicate possible child abuse in an injured child.

a. _____

b. _____

c. _____

d. _____

e. _____

67. What is the most critical aspect of nursing care of the pediatric trauma patient? _____

_____

Ingestions and Poisonings

68. Most poisonings occur as a result of _____.

69. Give the four methods used for removal of toxic substances.

a. _____

b. _____

c. _____

d. _____

70. Why does the American Academy of Pediatrics no longer recommend the use of syrup of ipecac in the home setting?

_____

_____

71. List three questions a nurse should ask the caregiver after a child has ingested a poisonous substance.

a. _____

b. _____

c. _____

Environmental Emergencies

72. List four local signs and symptoms of a snake bite.

a. _____

b. _____

c. _____

d. _____

73. Describe the nursing care of an injury from a dog bite. _____

_____

_____

Submersion Injuries

74. The injury to organ systems that occurs in a submersion injury is the result of _____.

75. Explain the relationship between submersion in cold water and the diving reflex.

_____

_____

76. Assessment of the child with a submersion injury focuses on which body system? _____

_____

77. Research studies have identified some of the needs of families of critically ill children. Name three.

a. _____

b. _____

c. _____

Heat-Related Emergencies

78. In all pediatric heat-related illnesses, the first priority is to _____.

79. Describe the treatment for heat exhaustion. _____

_____

80. What are the clinical manifestations of heat stroke? _____

_____

Dental Emergencies

Answer as either true (T) or false (F).

81. _____ In subluxation, the socket of the injured tooth is damaged.

82. _____ Intrusion of a tooth causes injury to the socket and underlying structures.

83. _____ An avulsed tooth should be placed in alcohol for transport to emergency care.

SUGGESTED LEARNING ACTIVITY

1. Observe an emergency department that handles pediatric clients. Ask the nurses about the kinds of pediatric problems that are seen most often.

STUDENT LEARNING APPLICATIONS

Enhance your learning by discussing your answers with other students.

You are observing in the emergency department when paramedics bring in 6-year-old Lindsay. While at her grandmother's house, Lindsey ingested several aspirin tablets. The nurse was performing a primary survey on Lindsay when the child went into cardiac arrest. Her father arrived in the emergency department while the trauma team was giving Lindsay cardiopulmonary resuscitation. When the father was told about Lindsay's condition, he began sobbing and repeating, "Please don't let her die." The nurse replied, "Don't worry, we won't. Everything will be fine."

1. While Lindsay is being stabilized, what questions should be directed at Lindsay's grandmother?

2. How would the nurse explain the rationale behind gastric lavage and administration of activated charcoal after Lindsay has been stabilized?

3. What do you think about the nurse's response to Lindsay's father? Offer an alternative response.

4. How can the nurse be supportive of Lindsay's father and grandmother through this emergency situation?

REVIEW QUESTIONS

Choose the best answer.

1. Which medication is used to treat severe acidosis associated with cardiac arrest?
   a. Epinephrine
   b. Calcium chloride
   c. Sodium bicarbonate
   d. Atropine sulfate

2. Which nursing action might help a toddler feel more comfortable in the emergency department?
   a. Perform the most distressing procedures first.
   b. Distract the child by counting numbers.
   c. Give the child a reward for cooperative behavior.
   d. Allow the child to hold his favorite toy.

3. Which is assessed first in an initial triage assessment?
   a. Respiratory rate and effort
   b. Skin color and temperature
   c. Response to environment
   d. Heart rate and rhythm

4. When a child's breathing makes a high-pitched sound on inspiration, what term should the nurse use to identify this sound?
   a. Snoring
   b. Stridor
   c. Wheezing
   d. Crackles

5. What is one reason that a small child is at a greater risk than an adult for airway problems?
   a. The child's thicker, inflexible trachea can more easily obstruct the airway.
   b. Children under 3 years of age are obligate nose breathers.
   c. The child's airway is narrower and more easily obstructed by small amounts of mucus.
   d. The child's smaller tongue creates more space for foreign body obstruction.

6. Which vital sign finding indicates that a 5-year-old requires immediate attention?
   a. Systolic blood pressure of 80 mm Hg
   b. Diastolic blood pressure of 60 mm Hg
   c. Heart rate of 94 beats per minute
   d. Respiratory rate of 62 breaths per minute

7. Which finding in a 1-year-old with hypovolemic shock should be reported immediately?
   a. Lungs clear on auscultation
   b. Palpable peripheral pulses
   c. Moist mucous membranes
   d. Less responsive to painful stimuli

8. What is the most common form of distributive shock?
   a. Septic
   b. Hypovolemic
   c. Cardiogenic
   d. Anaphylactic

9. The primary focus of assessment of cardiovascular status in a child with multiple traumatic injuries is to identify:
   a. hypovolemia.
   b. septic shock.
   c. cardiac arrest.
   d. electrolyte imbalance.

10. What is an indicator of hypovolemic shock in a 2-month-old? *(Choose all that apply.)*
    a. Bulging anterior fontanel
    b. Capillary refill of less than 2 seconds
    c. Parental report of two wet diapers in past 24 hours
    d. Extremities cool to the touch
    e. Dry mucous membranes

11. When drowning occurs, injury to organ systems is the result of:
    a. hypoxia.
    b. respiratory acidosis.
    c. hypokalemia.
    d. hypoglycemia.

12. After a 10-year-old falls on his face, his mother notices that the upper central incisors are loose. What should she do?
    a. Remove the loose teeth and put them in a container of warm milk.
    b. Call the dentist and schedule an appointment within the week.
    c. Leave the teeth alone and call the dentist for an immediate appointment.
    d. Ask the child to wiggle the teeth loose while driving to the nearest emergency department.

13. Which vital sign is measured first in children?
    a. Temperature
    b. Pulse
    c. Respiratory rate
    d. Blood pressure

14. What is the first compensatory mechanism for decreased oxygenation in children?
    a. Tachycardia
    b. Hypotension
    c. Cyanosis
    d. Diminished breath sounds

15. The nurse is planning an in-service about distributive (septic) shock for a group of ICU nurses. What information should the nurse include in the in-service? *(Choose all that apply.)*
    a. An early sign of septic shock is vasodilation.
    b. An early sign of septic shock is cold, clammy skin.
    c. An early sign of septic shock is tachycardia.
    d. A late sign of septic shock is oliguria.
    e. A late sign of septic shock is cyanosis.
    f. A late sign of septic shock is hepatomegaly.

16. The nurse is instructing a group of pediatric nurses about the treatment for ingestion of a poisonous substance. Which statement made by one of the pediatric nurses indicates a correct understanding of the teaching?
    a. "If a child ingests a corrosive, gastric lavage should be performed with a dose of vitamin K and the child is put on a low-fat, low-carbohydrate diet."
    b. "If acetaminophen is ingested, *N*-acetylcysteine (Mucomyst) should be administered with IV fluids and the child is put on a sodium-restricted, high-calorie, high-protein diet."
    c. "If a child ingests a hydrocarbon, vomiting should be induced with glucose for hypoglycemia and oxygen is administered."
    d. If aspirin is ingested, syrup of ipecac should be administered with sodium bicarbonate and volume expanders."

11 The Ill Child in the Hospital and Other Care Settings

HELPFUL HINT

Review Chapters 4 through 8 on growth and development and Chapter 3 in your textbook.

STUDENT LEARNING EXERCISES

Definitions

Match each term with its definition.

1. _____ Denial

2. _____ Egocentric

3. _____ Regression

4. _____ Separation anxiety

5. _____ Situational crisis

6. _____ Therapeutic play

a. An unanticipated event that poses a threat to an individual's well-being
b. Guided play that promotes the child's psychosocial or psychological well-being
c. Distress and apprehension caused by being removed from parents, the home, or familiar surroundings
d. Preoccupation with one's own interests and needs
e. Defense mechanism in which unpleasant realities are kept out of conscious awareness
f. Defense mechanism in which conflict or frustration is resolved by returning to a behavior that was successful in earlier years

Settings of Care

7. List four settings in which the pediatric nurse can provide health care or illness care to children.

a. _____

b. _____

c. _____

d. _____

Answer as either true (T) or false (F).

8. _____ One role of the pediatric nurse in a hospital setting is that of tour guide.

9. _____ A child having an asthma episode may be admitted to the hospital for a 24-hour observation.

10. _____ Because of time constraints in an emergency setting, preparing a child for a procedure is not an important nursing action.

11. _____ Teaching the child and family is less of a concern in an outpatient facility than it is in an acute care setting.

12. _____ In a rehabilitative setting, nurses must balance nurturing the child with setting limits as the child learns to be more self-sufficient.

13. _____ The nurse working in a school-based clinic needs to be sensitive to parental concerns regarding sexuality issues.

14. _____ In a community clinic, the nurse integrates health promotion and primary prevention into acute care.

15. _____ In home care, the nurse serves as case manager and care coordinator.

Stressors Associated with Illness and Hospitalization

16. Identify four factors that influence a child's reaction to illness.

    a. _____

    b. _____

    c. _____

    d. _____

17. Separation anxiety is most significant in the _____ and _____ age-groups.

18. Describe behaviors associated with the three stages of separation anxiety.

    Protest: _____

    Despair: _____

    Detachment: _____

19. How can nurses help parents deal with their hospitalized child's regression?

    _____

    _____

20. How can nurses minimize disruption in a toddler's usual routines during hospitalization?

    _____

    _____

21. How can hospitalization intensify a preschooler's fear of injury?

    _____

    _____

22. What can the nurse do to promote a sense of control in the school-age child while he or she is hospitalized?

    _____

    _____

23. Why is it important to provide hospitalized adolescents the opportunity to meet and interact with each other?

    _____

    _____

24. Give two examples of regressive behavior the nurse might observe in a child who is hospitalized.

   a. _____

   b. _____

Factors Affecting a Child's Response to Illness and Hospitalization

25. Identify three factors that affect how a child copes with illness or hospitalization.

   a. _____

   b. _____

   c. _____

26. Give two strategies that might facilitate a child's ability to cope with illness and hospitalization.

   a. _____

   b. _____

27. Identify two potential psychological benefits of hospitalization.

   a. _____

   b. _____

Playrooms in Health Care Settings

28. How is therapeutic play different from normal play? _____

   _____

29. What is emotional outlet play? _____

   _____

30. How can the nurse ensure the hospital playroom is a place where the child feels safe?

   _____

   _____

31. Give an example of how a child's cooperation with a treatment plan can be enhanced through play.

   _____

   _____

Chapter **11** The Ill Child in the Hospital and Other Care Settings

Admitting the Child to a Hospital Setting

32. How can the nurse set a positive tone for the child and family upon admission?

_____

_____

33. What is more important than completing the admission paperwork when the child is admitted to the hospital?

_____

_____

The Ill Child's Family

34. How does the role of the parent change when a child is hospitalized?

_____

_____

35. Identify three typical reactions that a child might have when a sibling is hospitalized.

a. _____

b. _____

c. _____

Developmental Approaches to the Hospitalized Child

Match each intervention with the appropriate age-group. Each age-group may be used more than once.

36. _____ It is important to follow home routines and rituals for this child.

37. _____ Provide a special area for activities for this child.

38. _____ Provide safe outlets for acting out aggression, such as painting and using play dough for this child.

39. _____ Reassure this child that he or she did not cause the illness.

40. _____ Assist this child in contacting friends.

41. _____ Limit the number of caregivers assigned to this child.

42. _____ Provide opportunities for non-nutritive sucking and oral stimulation for this child.

a. Neonate
b. Infant
c. Toddler
d. Preschooler
e. School-age children
f. Adolescent

SUGGESTED LEARNING ACTIVITIES

1. Observe a nurse in a school or community clinic, pediatrician's office, home care setting, or some other non-acute care setting. Compare the role of the pediatric nurse in this setting with that of the pediatric nurse in the hospital.

2. Develop a plan for a hospitalized toddler suffering from separation anxiety.

STUDENT LEARNING APPLICATIONS

Enhance your learning by discussing your answers with other students.

David is a 3-year-old who had an emergency appendectomy late last night. David has never been hospitalized before. David's mother is with him now. His father left to go to work after David came out of anesthesia, but he will return to the hospital after work. The family lives about an hour away from the hospital. David has a 7-year-old sister, Sara, who is in second grade; David's grandmother is taking care of Sara today.

1. What stressors do you think the family is experiencing at this time?

2. When you get a report on David, you learn that he clings to his mother every time a hospital staff person comes into his room. How can you help David cope with his fears?

3. David's mother tells you that she will be going home tonight with her husband because she needs to make arrangements for Sara's care. She expresses how guilty she feels about leaving him. How can you be supportive of her and her decision?

4. When you ask David whether he wants to have his blood pressure taken, he says "No." What would you do?

5. David has cried inconsolably for 2 hours since his parents left. When you go to check on him, you find that he has wet his pajamas. What is your interpretation of these behaviors? How would you explain them to David's mother when she calls to check on him?

6. What would be important to convey in your report to the nurse replacing you on the following shift?

REVIEW QUESTIONS

Choose the best answer.

1. Which child is most likely to have difficulty with separation anxiety during hospitalization?
   a. A 3-month-old
   b. An 18-month-old
   c. A 4-year-old
   d. A 7-year-old

2. Which type of behavior would you expect from a child in the denial stage of separation?
   a. Agitated
   b. Playful
   c. Withdrawn
   d. Anxious

3. A young child cries, kicks, and clings to his mother when she tries to leave. What is the nurse's best comment to the mother about this behavior?
   a. "This child is experiencing ineffective coping."
   b. "Parents should not leave their children when they are hospitalized."
   c. "Wait until the child falls asleep to leave."
   d. "This behavior actually shows a healthy attachment between you and your child."

4. Which would not be developmentally appropriate for a hospitalized adolescent?
   a. Allowing the adolescent to wear his or her own clothing.
   b. Providing privacy when giving treatments.
   c. Suggesting that his or her parents bring in his or her favorite foods.
   d. Discouraging visits from school friends.

5. Which nursing intervention might help the hospitalized toddler feel a sense of security and control?
   a. Follow the child's usual bedtime routine.
   b. Place the child in a crib with a cover over it.
   c. Tell the child what needs to be done and do not offer choices.
   d. Suggest to the parents that they bring new toys to the child.

Chapter **11** The Ill Child in the Hospital and Other Care Settings

6. What is the best response to a father who is concerned that his 4-year-old daughter, who has used the bathroom independently for more than a year now, has had a few accidents since being hospitalized?
   a. Suggest that he take his daughter to the bathroom more often.
   b. Assure him that this behavior will disappear immediately after discharge.
   c. Explain that children often exhibit regressive behaviors because of the stress of hospitalization.
   d. Set up a reward system to motivate the child to use the bathroom.

7. A 7-year-old who is scheduled to have a lumbar puncture tells the nurse, "I'm really nervous about this test." What is the best way for the nurse to minimize the child's anxiety about the procedure?
   a. Review the lumbar puncture procedure with him.
   b. Give him a relaxation tape with techniques to practice.
   c. Read a book to him about being in the hospital.
   d. Distract him by playing his favorite board game with him.

8. Ten-year-old Meg told the school nurse that she is worried about her twin sister, Mary, who is in the hospital. What might increase Meg's stress about her sister?
   a. Meg's grandparents are helping to care for her at home.
   b. Meg's parents have explained Mary's illness to her.
   c. Meg wonders whether she will get sick too.
   d. Meg plans to call her sister on the phone after school.

9. Emotional outlet play would be appropriate in which situation?
   a. A child who does not feel well enough to play
   b. A child who is having a hip spica cast applied in the morning
   c. A child who is scheduled for surgery next week
   d. A child who has been physically abused

10. Why might a 4-year-old child think that she caused the illness that resulted in her younger sibling being hospitalized?
    a. Preschool-age children understand disease transmission.
    b. The child feels insecure since the birth of the sibling.
    c. The feeling of closeness to her sibling makes her feel responsible for the illness.
    d. Children use magical thinking at this age.

11. The nurse is preparing an in-service for a group of new pediatric nurses about nursing care guidelines for siblings of an ill child. What information should the nurse include?
    a. Schedule limited time for the siblings to talk on the telephone.
    b. Encourage the ill child to discuss the experience of the illness or accident.
    c. Persuade the sibling to talk about only good events happening at home or school.
    d. Plan for the siblings to visit when the ill child is sleeping or at a procedure.

12. The nurse is caring for an 11-year-old child who will be hospitalized for at least 2 weeks following a motor vehicle accident. Which developmentally appropriate approach(es) should the nurse take when caring for the child? *(Choose all that apply.)*
    a. Encourage the child to assist in keeping the room in order.
    b. Encourage limited contact with friends.
    c. Involve the child in planning care for the day.
    d. Expect egocentric behavior.
    e. Accept regression but encourage independence.
    f. Set limits for behavior but allow for flexibility.

13. The nurse is talking to a parent of a 10-month-old who is in the hospital with respiratory syncytial virus. Which statement made by the parent would require the nurse to follow up?
    a. "I should bring in my baby's favorite blanket to provide security."
    b. "I know I can sleep in my baby's room, but I also need to go home to see my other children."
    c. "I should be present during procedures to help calm my baby."
    d. "I know I cannot help with the care of my baby but I wish I could give him a bath."

12 The Child with a Chronic Condition or Terminal Illness

Review Elizabeth Kübler-Ross' work on death and dying. You might also find it helpful to review concepts presented in Chapters 3, 4, and 11 of your textbook.

STUDENT LEARNING EXERCISES

Definitions

Match each term with its definition.

1. _____ Anticipatory grief

2. _____ Chronic grief

3. _____ Chronic condition

4. _____ Chronic sorrow

5. _____ Illness trajectory

6. _____ Hospice care

7. _____ Normalization

8. _____ Palliative care

a. The course of an illness
b. Responses used to counteract an illness or abnormal behavior in order to maintain appropriate and valued social roles
c. A system of comprehensive care that provides support and assistance to clients and families affected by terminal illness
d. An excessively long period of mourning that interferes with a person's ability to resume normal living
e. Recurrent feelings of grief, loss, and fear related to the child's illness and the loss of the ideal, healthy child
f. The processes of mourning, coping, interacting, planning, and psychosocial reorganization that occur as part of the response to the impending death of a loved one
g. Medical treatment or procedures that promote comfort and quality of life, rather than aiming to cure the underlying disease
h. A condition or illness that is long term and either without cure or with a residual effect that limits activities of daily living

9. In what ways has the experience of childhood chronic illness changed? _____

_____

_____

10. What does the phrase *children with special health care needs* mean? _____

_____

_____

The Family of the Child with Special Health Care Needs

11. What does the phrase *situational crisis* mean? _____

_____

_____

12. The predominant trait exhibited by resilient families is _____.

13. List four processes that enhance a family's resilience.

    a. _____

    b. _____

    c. _____

    d. _____

Answer as either true (T) or false (F).

14. _____ In resilient families, the child's condition-related needs become the focus around which family activities revolve.

15. _____ For resilient families, coping is an active process that involves learning about their child's condition and available resources.

The Grieving Process

16. The nurse caring for a child with a chronic illness must keep in mind that the most important aspect of a chronic illness is that it affects _____

    _____.

17. Identify the five stages of the grieving process delineated by Kübler-Ross.

    a. _____

    b. _____

    c. _____

    d. _____

    e. _____

Answer as either true (T) or false (F).

18. _____ Children move through the five stages of the grieving process sequentially.

19. _____ Children with chronic conditions use denial more frequently than adults.

The Child with Special Health Care Needs

20. Children's responses to illness are influenced by their _____ and their _____.

21. Nurses caring for children with chronic conditions must understand issues concerning _____ and _____ in relation to each stage of growth and development.

Answer as either true (T) or false (F).

22. _____ Temporary regression may be observed in children of all ages.

23. _____ Raising a child with a chronic illness necessitates that parents learn a different set of child-rearing techniques.

The Child with a Chronic Illness

24. The goals for a child with a chronic illness are:

a. _____

b. _____

25. The goals for the entire family are:

a. _____

b. _____

c. _____

26. What is the first factor the nurse must consider when planning care for a child with a chronic illness?

_____.

27. _____ is the most important factor in establishing a good relationship with a child and family.

Answer as either true (T) or false (F).

28. _____ The expression of emotions is always better than holding emotions inside.

29. _____ Honesty and trust must be maintained at all times when caring for a child with a chronic condition.

30. _____ Siblings of a chronically ill child may use regression as a coping mechanism.

31. _____ Siblings should not participate in the ill child's physical care.

The Terminally Ill or Dying Child

Match each age group with the corresponding concept of death.

32. _____ Infants/toddlers

33. _____ Early childhood

34. _____ Middle childhood

35. _____ Adolescents

a. Death is temporary and reversible.
b. Death is a sad and irreversible event.
c. Death is viewed as the loss of a caretaker.
d. Death is inevitable and irreversible.

Answer as either true (T) or false (F).

36. _____ One of the primary concerns of dying children is the fear of being alone.

37. _____ It is unusual for parents to talk about the experience of the child's illness and death.

38. _____ An important aspect of supporting the sibling of a child who has died is to acknowledge that the loss is significant.

39. Identify three self-care measures that can assist nurses caring for terminally ill children.

    a. _____

    b. _____

    c. _____

40. What is the most common issue surrounding a child's impending death? _____

    _____

    _____

Answer as either true (T) or false (F).

41. _____ Pain control is often the most troubling concern for dying children, family, and nursing staff.

42. _____ Hospice care for terminally ill children is increasing.

43. _____ The nurse should provide privacy for the dying child and family.

44. _____ Adequate oral intake is crucial to the dying child's comfort.

45. _____ Hearing is the last sense to cease before death.

46. _____ The young child is usually not aware of the presence of parents during the dying process.

47. _____ Respiratory changes are always the earliest indicators of imminent death.

48. _____ Hypercapnia has a sedative effect.

49. _____ The nurse's response to caring for a dying child will correlate to a certain degree with the Kübler-Ross stages of grieving.

50. _____ Nurses with many years of experience in caring for dying children will typically not feel grief when a child dies.

SUGGESTED LEARNING ACTIVITIES

1. Investigate the availability of pediatric hospice care in your area.

2. Make a home visit to the family of a child with a chronic illness. How does home care compare with hospital care?

STUDENT LEARNING APPLICATIONS

Enhance your learning by discussing your answers with other students.

1. What are your fears or concerns about caring for a child who is dying? Talk with other students about your thoughts. Are your fears or concerns similar or different from those of the other students?

2. Talk to a nurse who has worked with dying children and their families. What was the most rewarding aspect of this work? What was the most difficult? Share what you learned with other students.

Choose the best answer.

1. The most significant concern of the parents of a dying child is the child's:
   a. pain.
   b. hydration.
   c. safety.
   d. privacy.

2. A 5-year-old understands death as:
   a. the loss of a caretaker.
   b. a temporary separation.
   c. sad and permanent.
   d. something that happens to everyone.

3. Although an individual may fluctuate between stages of the grieving process, the first stage is usually:
   a. denial.
   b. resentment.
   c. bargaining.
   d. depression.

4. Chronic illness with frequent hospitalizations can affect the psychosocial development of a school-age child by:
   a. leading to feelings of inferiority.
   b. interfering with developing a sense of initiative.
   c. interfering with parental attachment.
   d. blocking the development of identity.

5. What is the best response to an adolescent who asks whether he should talk to his dying brother?
   a. "You might want to hold his hand instead because he cannot hear you."
   b. "Although he may not answer you, your brother can still hear what you are saying."
   c. "He can't hear you but he can feel your presence nearby."
   d. "Talk about happy things because you don't want to upset him."

6. What is a trait of resilient families?
   a. Disengaging the family from the community
   b. Maintaining rigid family roles
   c. Engaging in efforts to keep the family intact
   d. Focusing on the child's condition-related needs

7. What interventions are appropriate when caring for a chronically ill toddler? *(Choose all that apply.)*
   a. Prepare for procedures days in advance.
   b. Arrange for friends to visit in the hospital.
   c. Limit parent participation in the child's care.
   d. Keep security objects nearby.
   e. Provide opportunities for play.
   f. Maintain consistent limits.

8. What is the nurse's first consideration when planning care for the child with a chronic illness?
   a. Child's condition
   b. Child's development
   c. Family's coping mechanisms
   d. Family's understanding of prognosis

Chapter **12** **The Child with a Chronic Condition or Terminal Illness**

9. The nurse is preparing an in-service about nursing care for a dying child and the family. What information should be included in the teaching?
   a. The nurse should impose his or her personal beliefs to help the family with the grieving process.
   b. The amount of time a family spends with the child after death should be limited to allow the family to start making arrangements.
   c. The nurse should allow the family to talk about the child's illness and death to help with the grieving process.
   d. The nurse should not allow the siblings of the dying child to stay in the room when death is imminent to avoid scaring the siblings.

10. Which things enhance the family's resilience when caring for a child with a chronic illness? *(Choose all that apply.)*
    a. Improved technology
    b. Families are reimbursed
    c. Maintaining open communication
    d. Preserving family boundaries
    e. Allocating health care resources
    f. Establishing community resources

13 Principles and Procedures for Nursing Care of Children

HELPFUL HINT

Review Chapters 3 and 11 of your textbook.

STUDENT LEARNING EXERCISES

Definitions

Match each term with its correct definition.

1. _____ Informed consent

2. _____ Apical pulse rate

3. _____ Enteral

4. _____ Antipyretic

5. _____ Auscultate

6. _____ Lavage

a. To listen to body sounds
b. By way of the digestive system
c. Requirement that both the child and the parent/guardian completely understand the proposed procedures or treatments
d. An agent that reduces or relieves fever
e. Process of washing out or irrigating an organ
f. Heart rate determined by placing stethoscope over the PMI and counting for 1 minute

Preparing Children for Procedures

7. List five assessments the nurse should make in preparing a child and family for an invasive procedure.

a. _____

b. _____

c. _____

d. _____

e. _____

Answer as either true (T) or false (F).

8. _____ Children need to be prepared before any procedure is performed.

9. _____ Parents need to be prepared before a procedure is performed on their child.

10. _____ It is preferable to perform painful or invasive procedures in the treatment room.

11. _____ The nurse should only praise children when they have been cooperative during a procedure.

12. _____ Parents should be asked to step out of the room before an invasive procedure is started.

13. _____ Informed consent is obtained from the parent before any surgical or diagnostic invasive procedures.

14. _____ Children older than age 7 years can give informed consent for procedures.

77

Transporting Infants and Children

15. Name four factors that must be considered when choosing the method of transportation for a hospitalized child.

a. _____

b. _____

c. _____

d. _____

Using Restraints

Answer as either true (T) or false (F).

16. _____ All possible alternatives to restraint should be considered before the restraint is applied.

17. _____ The physician's order for restraints should indicate why the restraints are necessary and how long they should be in place.

18. _____ When restraints are applied, the extremities distal to the restraints are assessed for temperature, pulses, and capillary refill.

19. _____ Restraints should be removed every 4 hours for range-of-motion exercises and repositioning.

Infection Control

20. List the four body components to which standard precautions apply.

a. _____

b. _____

c. _____

d. _____

21. Second-tier precautions are also called _____.

22. Describe how to use an alcohol-based rub. _____

_____

_____

Bathing Infants and Children

23. The temperature of water used to bathe a child should not exceed _____.

24. If a thermometer is not accessible, the nurse can determine whether water temperature is comfortable by

_____.

25. When bathing an infant in the tub, the nurse makes sure that the water level does not exceed _____ inches.

26. What is the rationale for avoiding talcum powder after a child's bath? _____

_____

Oral Hygiene

Answer as either true (T) or false (F).

27. _____ Young children require supervision while brushing their teeth.

28. _____ A quarter-sized amount of toothpaste should be placed on the toothbrush each time the child brushes his
or her teeth.

29. _____ Avoid cleaning the teeth when the child is at risk for gingival bleeding.

Feeding

30. What is the rationale for not propping up a bottle when feeding an infant? _____

_____

31. Name three strategies that might make hospital meals more desirable for young children.

a. _____

b. _____

c. _____

Vital Signs

32. What are the indications for measuring axillary temperatures in children? _____

_____

33. What factors might cause an inaccurate measurement of oral temperature? _____

_____

34. The nurse should take a child's apical pulse if the child:

a. _____

b. _____

c. _____

35. How long should the nurse count a heart rate when measuring an apical pulse? _____

36. The nurse measuring respirations on a 6-month-old would auscultate breath sounds for _____ seconds.

37. The nurse measuring blood pressure hears a systolic pressure at 88 mm Hg and continues to hear it down to a

measurement of 0 mm Hg. This blood pressure should be recorded as _____.

Chapter **13** **Principles and Procedures for Nursing Care of Children**

Fever-Reducing Measures

38. List two environmental measures that can be taken to treat a child's fever.

    a. _____

    b. _____

39. The generic names of drugs used to treat fever in children are _____ and _____.

Specimen Collection

40. Regardless of the type of specimen to be obtained, the nurse should use _____ precautions.

41. The technique used for obtaining a sample of an infant's nasopharyngeal secretions is _____.

42. Catheterization at home is usually performed as a _____ procedure.

43. The most common site for bone marrow aspiration in a child is the _____.

Gavage and Gastrostomy

44. When and how often should the nurse check placement of a nasogastric tube? _____

    _____

45. Name three methods for determining placement of a nasogastric tube.

    a. _____

    b. _____

    c. _____

Answer as either true (T) or false (F).

46. _____ The most reliable method for determining nasogastric tube placement is auscultation of air entering the stomach.

47. _____ Tube placement and residual volumes should be checked every 24 hours when continuous enteral feedings are infusing.

48. _____ The only definitive method of determining the correct position of a feeding tube is radiographic confirmation.

49. _____ When a bolus feeding is completed, the child is placed on the left side for 30 minutes.

Enemas

50. When giving an enema to a 7-year-old, the nurse should use a volume of _____ mL and insert the tube into the rectum to a depth of _____ inches.

Care of Ostomies

Answer as either true (T) or false (F).

51. _____ The consistency of stool through an ostomy is determined by the anatomic location of the stoma.

52. _____ The nursing care of a child with an ostomy differs very little from that of an adult.

Oxygen Therapy

53. How does oxygen therapy in children differ from therapy in adults? _____

_____

Assessing Oxygenation

54. The nurse measures a child's pulse oximetry to be 98%. What does this finding indicate?

_____

55. What action should the nurse take if this child's pulse oximetry drops to 89%?

_____

Tracheostomy Care

56. What are the five elements of routine tracheostomy care?

a. _____

b. _____

c. _____

d. _____

e. _____

57. How often should the nurse perform tracheostomy care? _____

58. Catheter insertion and suctioning time should be limited to _____.

59. The suction catheter is inserted with the suction _____.

Surgical Procedures

60. At what point preoperatively should clear liquids be stopped? _____

_____

61. What nursing interventions are appropriate to prevent atelectasis postoperatively?

_____

_____

Chapter **13** **Principles and Procedures for Nursing Care of Children**

62. Identify five stressors that may be experienced by a child undergoing surgery.

a. _____

b. _____

c. _____

d. _____

e. _____

SUGGESTED LEARNING ACTIVITY

1. Follow a child through a surgical experience. Take note of preoperative procedures, teaching, and postanesthesia care. When the child returns to the unit, provide immediate postoperative care. Describe the similarities and differences in preoperative and postoperative nursing care for a child compared with the care of an adult.

STUDENT LEARNING APPLICATIONS

Enhance your learning by discussing your answers with other students.

Betsy is a 3-year-old who is scheduled for surgery in the morning. She and her parents have just arrived at her assigned room, and you are assigned to admit Betsy to the unit. Betsy's admission orders include routine urinalysis and complete blood cell count.

1. How are you going to measure Betsy's vital signs?

2. Betsy is not toilet trained yet. How would you collect a urine specimen from her?

3. Her mother tells you that she wants to stay with Betsy when you take blood for the CBC. What is your response? Where are you planning to do this procedure?

4. How would you explain the procedure for venipuncture to Betsy?

5. Betsy's father wants to know when she has to stop eating before surgery. What would you tell him?

6. What information do you want to get from Betsy and her parents before you do any preoperative teaching?

REVIEW QUESTIONS

Choose the correct answer.

1. A parent wants to wait outside until a procedure is completed on his child. What would be the nurse's best response?
   a. "It would be better for your child if you were by his side."
   b. "That is fine. I will stay with your child during the procedure."
   c. "It is hospital policy for parents to step out of the room during procedures."
   d. "This test will only take a few minutes. Why don't you stay?"

2. What temperature indicates fever?
   a. Rectal temperature of 100.6° F
   b. Rectal temperature of 99.5° F
   c. Oral temperature of 98.9° F
   d. Axillary temperature of 97.9° F

3. What should the nurse suggest that parents do to reduce their child's fever?
   a. Give the child an alcohol bath.
   b. Give the child a sponge bath in tepid water.
   c. Administer baby aspirin.
   d. Dress the child in heavy-weight clothing.

4. What is the best indicator that the nurse is correctly measuring vital signs on an infant?
   a. Measuring oral temperature for 5 minutes
   b. Counting apical pulse for 60 seconds
   c. Recording respiratory rate from the cardiorespiratory monitor
   d. Recording blood pressure as P/46

5. A 9-year-old asks the nurse where the doctor is going to put the needle for the bone marrow test. The nurse describes the location as the:
   a. lower middle part of his back.
   b. middle part of his chest.
   c. right or left side of his hip.
   d. top bone in his leg.

6. When an extremity is restrained, it is essential for the nurse to assess the affected area for:
   a. clubbing.
   b. pallor.
   c. spasm.
   d. crepitus.

7. Nasogastric tube placement should be checked:
   a. before initiating a bolus feeding.
   b. when the feeding is completed.
   c. every 12 hours during continuous feedings.
   d. when residual volumes are excessive.

8. The nurse should discontinue a bolus gavage feeding if which of the following occurs?
   a. Fatigue
   b. Crying
   c. Phlebitis
   d. Vomiting

9. Which statement about ostomies is correct?
   a. The lower the stoma along the intestinal tract, the more liquid the stool.
   b. Urinary stomas do not begin to drain until the second postoperative day.
   c. A minimal amount of drainage from colostomies is normal up to four days after surgery.
   d. Children usually do not require appliances on their stomas.

10. A 2-year-old is scheduled for surgery tomorrow. The parents have been told to arrive at the short-procedure unit at 8 AM. The nurse should expect preoperative feeding instructions to include:
    a. clear liquids until midnight tonight and then nothing by mouth.
    b. stopping solid food at 5 AM and then clear liquids until 7 AM.
    c. fluids including milk and orange juice until arrival at the hospital.
    d. clear liquids until 6 AM and then nothing to eat or drink.

Chapter **13** **Principles and Procedures for Nursing Care of Children**

11. The nurse is caring for an 8-month-old who needs a nasogastric tube placed for continuous feedings. Place in correct order the sequence of steps for placing a nasogastric tube in an infant.
   a. Measure the distance from the tip of the nose to the earlobe and midpoint between the end of the xiphoid and the umbilicus.
   b. Aspirate the gastric contents and perform pH testing.
   c. Lubricate the tube with water-soluble lubricant.
   d. Position the infant on the back or right side.
   e. Insert tube gently but firmly toward the back of the throat.
   f. Secure the tube with tape.

12. The nurse is teaching a parent of a 4-year-old child how to perform intermittent feedings at home. Which statement made by the parent would indicate a correct understanding of how to perform the procedure?
   a. "I should have the head of the bed flat while my child is receiving the nasogastric feeding."
   b. "I should flush the nasogastric tube with sterile water after the feeding is completed."
   c. "I should check the placement of the nasogastric tube only if there is a residual."
   d. "I should use cold formula for the nasogastric feeding that will flow slowly over 30 minutes."

13. The nurse caring for an 8-year-old girl needs to obtain a sterile urine sample. Which action(s) will the nurse expect to take while performing the catheterization? *(Choose all that apply.)*
   a. Encourage the child to hold her breath during the procedure.
   b. Tell the child to bear down to relax the external sphincter.
   c. Direct the catheter slightly upward when inserting the catheter.
   d. Insert the catheter another inch once urine is observed.
   e. Collect the urine in a sterile specimen cup.

14 Medication Administration and Safety for Infants and Children

HELPFUL HINT

Review pharmacodynamics and pharmacokinetics in a pharmacology or nursing fundamentals textbook.

STUDENT LEARNING EXERCISES

Definitions

Match each term with its definition.

1. _____ Eutectic mixture of local anesthetics

2. _____ Metered-dose inhaler

3. _____ Pharmacodynamics

4. _____ Pharmacokinetics

5. _____ Central venous access device

6. _____ Peripherally inserted central line

a. Central line inserted through the antecubital vein into the superior vena cava
b. Hand-held device that delivers "puffs" of medication for inhalation
c. Cream used to numb skin at a depth of 0.5 mm
d. Behavior of medications at the cellular level
e. Catheter tip placed in the superior vena cava
f. Time and movement relationships of medications

Pharmacokinetics in Children

7. Name four factors that influence absorption of medications administered orally.

   a. _____

   b. _____

   c. _____

   d. _____

Answer as either true (T) or false (F).

8. _____ Infants have a larger body surface area in proportion to their weight compared with adults.

9. _____ Compared with an adult, a child requires a lower dose per kilogram of a water-soluble medication to achieve its desired effect.

10. _____ The immaturity of the blood-brain barrier in a child results in a decreased distribution of medications to the brain.

11. What factors affect drug excretion in the infant? _____

_____

Chapter **14** **Medication Administration and Safety for Infants and Children**

12. Why would a peak and trough serum level be measured? _____

_____

13. The level at which the serum concentration is lowest is referred to as the medication _____.

Psychological and Developmental Differences

14. Name three ways parents can assist the nurse with administering medications to children.

    a. _____

    b. _____

    c. _____

15. Describe two strategies to elicit cooperation from children of the following age-groups when administering medications to them.

    Toddler:

    a. _____

    b. _____

    Preschooler:

    a. _____

    b. _____

    School-age child:

    a. _____

    b. _____

Calculating Dosages

Answer as either true (T) or false (F).

16. _____ Standard doses exist for pediatric medications.

17. _____ Pediatric doses are usually calculated on the basis of the child's weight in pounds.

18. _____ The most reliable method for determining pediatric medication dosages is to use the body surface area formula.

Administration Procedures

19. List three procedures that should be followed to avoid medication errors when medications are given to children.

    a. _____

    b. _____

    c. _____

20. Why is the oral route one of the least reliable methods for medication administration?

_____

_____

21. What should a nurse do if a child cannot swallow tablets or capsules?

_____

_____

22. Why should the nurse mix a powdered medication with a "nonessential" food?

_____

_____

Medication Administration

Answer as either true (T) or (F) false.

23. _____ Honey can be mixed with medications and given to infants.

24. _____ A sustained-release tablet can be crushed if the child cannot swallow it.

25. _____ Medication should be placed in the child's mouth along the side of the cheek.

26. _____ Oral medications should be administered with the child in an upright position.

27. How can the nurse hold a 3-year-old child who does not want to take his or her medication?

_____

_____

28. What nursing action should be taken if a child vomits his or her medication 15 minutes after it was given?

_____

_____

29. What procedures should be followed when medications are administered through a feeding tube?

_____

_____

Administering Injections

30. What are the guidelines for giving an explanation to a child before an injection is administered?

_____

_____

Chapter **14** **Medication Administration and Safety for Infants and Children**

31. What can the nurse do to make injections less painful? _____

_____

Administering Intramuscular Injections

Match each injection site with its indication for use.

32. _____ Vastus lateralis   a. Not used for young children because muscle cannot hold the volume of medication

33. _____ Ventrogluteal   b. Usually used for children younger than 3 years of age

                                      c. Safe for children older than 18 months

34. _____ Dorsogluteal   d. Not used until child has been walking for at least 1 year

35. _____ Deltoid

Answer as either true (T) or false (F).

36. _____ The nurse should document the site used for an injection.

37. _____ The air bubble technique should be used when preparing pediatric injections.

38. _____ Toddlers can receive up to 1.5 mL of a drug safely in the ventrogluteal site.

39. _____ Viscous medication is less painful when it is injected through a smaller-gauge needle.

Administering Subcutaneous Injections

40. A subcutaneous injection should not be used if _____ is impaired.

41. Name four areas of the body that are preferred subcutaneous injection sites.

     a. _____

     b. _____

     c. _____

     d. _____

Answer as either true (T) or false (F).

42. _____ Subcutaneous injection sites need to be rotated to prevent the development of abscesses.

43. _____ The angle of needle insertion for a subcutaneous injection is usually 90 degrees.

44. _____ Volumes for subcutaneous injections can be as high as 3 mL.

Intradermal Injections

45. The intradermal route is most often used for _____.

46. What sites are used for intradermal injections? _____

_____

47. Describe the procedure for administering an intradermal injection. _____

_____

Rectal and Vaginal Administration

Answer as either true (T) or false (F).

48. _____ The child should be placed in a prone position for administration of a rectal suppository.

49. _____ The nurse should direct the child to take a deep breath as medication is inserted into the rectum.

50. _____ The vaginal route is used to treat candidal infections.

Ophthalmic and Otic Administration

Answer as either true (T) or false (F).

51. _____ Instillation of ophthalmic drops is a sterile procedure.

52. _____ Otic solutions should be warmed to room temperature before being administered.

53. _____ To administer ear drops to a 5-year-old, pull the pinna of the ear down and back.

Inhalation Therapy

54. A _____ used with a metered-dose inhaler increases the effectiveness of the medication.

55. How long should a child hold their breath after inhaling a "puff" of medication from a metered-dose inhaler?

_____

Intravenous Therapy

56. What factors should be considered when selecting a site for an intravenous line?

_____

57. List a nonpharmacologic technique for helping a child cope with the discomfort of intravenous catheter insertion.

_____

58. What are the guidelines for using an eutectic mixture of local anesthetic cream before insertion of an intravenous catheter?

_____

_____

59. Why should a volumetric infusion pump be used when IV fluids are administered?

_____

60. How frequently should an IV site be assessed? _____

61. What assessments should be made? _____

62. The formula for calculating maintenance fluid needs is _____.

Chapter **14** **Medication Administration and Safety for Infants and Children**

63. Calculate the maintenance fluid requirements for children of the following weights:

35 kg: _____

16 kg: _____

64. What is meant by IV push medications? _____

_____

65. Why is it important to flush the IV tubing after an IV piggyback medication is administered? _____

_____

66. How frequently should an intermittent infusion port or heparin lock be flushed? _____

_____

67. In what types of situations are central venous access devices used? _____

_____

68. What is an implanted venous access device? _____

_____

69. The major complications of peripherally inserted central catheters (PICC lines) are _____

_____.

Administration of Blood or Blood Products

Answer as either true (T) or false (F).

70. _____ Blood should be infused with a dextrose solution on a piggyback setup.

71. _____ An important nursing action is to monitor the child's vital signs before and during a blood transfusion.

72. _____ The infusion is discontinued if a transfusion reaction is suspected.

Child and Family Education

73. List six points that need to be addressed when teaching parents about administering medications to a child at home.

a. _____

b. _____

c. _____

d. _____

e. _____

f. _____

SUGGESTED LEARNING ACTIVITY

1. Review a child's medication administration record. Calculate dosages for prescribed medications. Determine whether the prescribed dosage is safe for the child. Observe medication administration. What techniques were helpful to the child? To the nurse?

STUDENT LEARNING APPLICATIONS

Enhance your learning by discussing your answers with other students.

Kelly is a 9-year-old girl with cystic fibrosis. Kelly is in the hospital because of an exacerbation. Her cough has worsened, she has lost weight, and she is mildly dehydrated. Kelly weighs 55 pounds. Her admission orders include IV fluids and medications.

1. Kelly needs to have an IV placed for fluids and medications. What could you do to minimize her discomfort before and during the venipuncture?

2. There is an order to give Kelly D5.225 NSS at 65 mL/hr. Calculate her maintenance fluid requirements. How does this order compare with your calculation?

3. There is an order to give tobramycin 40 mg IVPB every 8 hours. The dosage range for children is 6 to 7.5 mg/kg/day divided every 8 hours. Is Kelly's dosage within that range?

4. Two days later Kelly's maintenance IV is converted to a heparin lock. How does the care of a heparin lock differ from that of a continuous IV?

5. Kelly's IV has infiltrated, and a PICC line is discussed. What is a PICC line? What are the advantages of having a PICC line instead of a heparin lock?

6. Kelly needs to take Pancrease (Ultrase MT) capsules before meals and snacks. Her mother tells you Kelly cannot swallow pills. What additional information would you want her to know about giving medications to Kelly?

7. When you approach Kelly to administer her oral medications, she turns her head away and puts her hand over her mouth. What would you do to get Kelly to take her medications? What would you do if Kelly's mother were present?

REVIEW QUESTIONS

Choose the best answer.

1. Physiologic differences in the gastrointestinal system between children and adults affect which component of drug action?
   a. Absorption
   b. Distribution
   c. Metabolism
   d. Excretion

2. Drug toxicity may occur more rapidly in the infant for which reason?
   a. Larger surface area requires a larger dosage.
   b. Fewer enzymes are available to bind with the drug.
   c. Renal immaturity may delay drug excretion.
   d. The blood-brain barrier becomes less selective with maturity.

3. The pediatric maintenance dosage for phenytoin (Dilantin) is 4 to 8 mg/kg/day in three equal doses. An acceptable dosage for a child weighing 15 kg is:
   a. 30 mg.
   b. 60 mg.
   c. 90 mg.
   d. 120 mg.

Chapter **14** **Medication Administration and Safety for Infants and Children**

4. Which food is the best choice for mixing with a medication to be administered to an infant?
   a. Honey
   b. Cherry syrup
   c. Similac with iron
   d. Pudding

5. Which site should the nurse use to administer an intramuscular injection to a 17-month-old?
   a. Deltoid
   b. Dorsogluteal
   c. Vastus lateralis
   d. Ventrogluteal

6. When administering insulin subcutaneously the nurse should:
   a. use a 1- to 1.5-inch needle.
   b. rotate injection sites.
   c. administer a very small volume such as 0.1 mL.
   d. inject the needle at a 30-degree angle.

7. Which action is appropriate for the administration of a rectal suppository?
   a. Position the child on his abdomen.
   b. Insert the suppository 1 to 2 inches.
   c. Direct the child to take a deep breath.
   d. Ask the child to get up and walk around after insertion.

8. Which statement about the administration of IV piggyback medications is correct?
   a. The undiluted medication is pushed directly into the IV catheter through the port closest to the patient.
   b. The medication is injected into the port nearest the child and flushed through the tubing slowly.
   c. The IV catheter is used intermittently when medication is infused over a 1- to 2-hour period.
   d. The medication is diluted in at least 20 mL of IV fluid and infused over at least 15 minutes.

9. Which action(s) should be taken before the nurse administers a medication to a 16-year-old? *(Choose all that apply.)*
   a. Adhere to the six rights of medication administration.
   b. Use oral, liquid medications for all children to ensure accurate dosing.
   c. Double check medication calculations before administration.
   d. Ask another RN to double check certain medications.
   e. Note the child's allergies.
   f. Use adult-specific concentrations that are re-concentrated for children.

10. A nurse is preparing to give a subcutaneous injection of insulin to a 9-year-old child. Place in correct order the sequence of steps for giving an intramuscular injection.
    a. Gently pinch the tissue to raise the subcutaneous tissue.
    b. Release the tissue and inject the medicine.
    c. Clean site in a circular motion with an antiseptic swab.
    d. Insert the needle using a dart-like motion.

11. The nurse is teaching a parent who needs to administer an antibiotic at home to a 5-year-old. Which statement made by the parent would indicate a need for additional teaching?
    a. "I should complete the full course of the antibiotic even if my child does not have a fever for longer than 24 hours."
    b. "I need to use a calibrated spoon or oral syringe to give the correct amount of the antibiotic to my child."
    c. "I can put the antibiotic into a food such as applesauce or a drink such as grape juice so my child will take the complete dose."
    d. "I can keep this antibiotic on the kitchen counter so that I remember to administer it to my child as scheduled."

15 Pain Management for Children

HELPFUL HINT

Review pain management in a medical-surgical nursing textbook.

STUDENT LEARNING EXERCISES

Definitions

Match each term with its definition.

1. _____ Addiction

2. _____ Adjuvant

3. _____ Epidural

4. _____ Nociceptive

5. _____ Pain

6. _____ Pain threshold

7. _____ Opioid

a. Natural or synthetic opium derivative used for analgesia
b. Impulse giving rise to the sensation of pain
c. Psychological and neurologic state of need for and compulsive use of drugs
d. Unpleasant sensory and emotional experience associated with actual or potential tissue damage
e. Situated within the spinal canal, on or outside the dura mater
f. Level of intensity at which pain becomes appreciable or perceptible
g. An intervention with additive effects on pain management designed to assist the primary pain management intervention

Definitions and Theories of Pain

8. According to McCaffrey and Pasero, *pain* is _____

_____.

9. The International Association for the Study of Pain defines *pain* as _____

_____.

Answer as either true (T) or false (F).

10. _____ The gate control theory supports the use of physiological and psychological interventions in pain management.

11. _____ Rubbing a sprained ankle makes the pain worse.

12. _____ A child with arthritis typically feels acute pain.

13. _____ Acute pain felt by hospitalized children is often procedural pain.

14. _____ Chronic pain affects a child's ability to lead a normal life.

Research on Pain in Children

15. A three-step ladder for treating cancer pain was developed by _____.

16. Guidelines for managing pain in sickle cell disease were developed by _____.

17. The _____ added new standards that integrate pain assessment and management into their accreditation standards.

Myths About Pain and Pain Management in Children

Answer as either true (T) or false (F).

18. _____ Myelinization is not necessary for pain perception.

19. _____ Emotional factors contribute to the pain experience.

20. _____ Children are at higher risk for respiratory depression from narcotics than are adults.

21. _____ Premature infants lack the neurologic capacity to feel pain.

22. _____ Infants cannot remember painful experiences.

Assessment of Pain in Children

23. To assess pain in infants, the nurse looks for _____ and _____ signs.

24. As infants get older, their responses to pain change from generalized to _____ responses.

25. It is important for the nurse to distinguish between pain and _____ in infants.

26. Toddlers may react to pain with generalized _____.

27. Preschoolers may think that pain is a _____.

28. Give two reasons why a school-age child might overreact to pain.

    a. _____

    b. _____

29. How may adolescent egocentrism affect how they communicate about pain?

    _____

    _____

30. Why is it imperative to use pain assessment tools with children?

    _____

    _____

31. Pain self-report tools are usually appropriate for children older than _____ years.

32. Which pain assessment tools use a photographic scale and a numeric scale?

_____

_____

Non-Pharmacologic and Pharmacologic Pain Interventions

33. What are the benefits of regulated breathing techniques? _____

_____

34. Explain how children who are using distraction are not necessarily pain free. _____

_____

35. Guided imagery involves _____ and _____.

36. What is biofeedback? _____

_____

37. What are the benefits of progressive muscle relaxation in older children? _____

_____

38. What is hypnosis? _____

_____

39. A TENS unit interferes with the _____.

40. For children receiving patient-controlled analgesia therapy, the following items should be readily available:

a. _____

b. _____

c. _____

41. If naloxone is administered too rapidly, _____ may result.

Answer as either true (T) or false (F).

42. _____ Topical anesthetic creams are used as numbing agents.

43. _____ Nonsteroidal antiinflammatory drugs (NSAIDs) reduce pain and inflammation.

44. _____ Acetaminophen does not inhibit prostaglandin.

45. _____ Opioid analgesics can cause sedation and respiratory depression.

46. _____ Meperidine (Demerol) is a more effective analgesic than morphine in children.

47. _____ Midazolam (Versed) is used for conscious sedation.

48. _____ Epidural analgesics have fewer side effects than opioid analgesics.

Chapter **15** **Pain Management for Children**

SUGGESTED LEARNING ACTIVITIES

1. Interview a pediatric nurse about his or her experiences with managing pain in children. Discover how the nurse assesses pain in children who have chronic pain. Ask the nurse to explain how he or she designs a plan for managing chronic pain in children.

2. Interview the parent of an infant or toddler. Discover how the parent knows that the child is in pain.

STUDENT LEARNING APPLICATIONS

Enhance your learning by discussing your answers with other students.

Jose, an 8-year-old boy who weighs 30 kg, is experiencing acute pain. The physician orders 3 mg of morphine sulfate IV every 4 hours for pain. Jose receives 3 mg at 9 AM. At 9:30 AM, he rates his pain as 0 on a 0 to 5 rating scale. At noon, he complains of "bad pain" and rates his pain as 5 on the same scale.

1. What do you think about Jose's order for pain medication? What changes may be required?

2. What other questions would you ask Jose about his pain?

3. What questions would you ask Jose about what else might be helpful in managing his pain?

4. How would you present your findings to Jose's physician?

REVIEW QUESTIONS

Choose the best answer.

1. The best indicator of pain in a 15-month-old toddler is:
   a. behavioral changes.
   b. changes in vital signs.
   c. parental assessment.
   d. child's verbal response.

2. Which are the side effects of opioid analgesics? *(Choose all that apply.)*
   a. Constipation
   b. Excessive thirst
   c. Sedation
   d. Nausea
   e. Muscle weakness

3. A hospitalized 12-year-old is playing Nintendo and rates her pain as 1 on a 0 to 5 rating scale. This activity is an example of:
   a. imagery.
   b. distraction.
   c. play therapy.
   d. self-hypnosis.

4. A child's perception of pain is influenced by:
   a. the parent's response to the child's pain.
   b. the child's cultural background.
   c. the child's developmental stage.
   d. all of the above.

5. Postoperative pain is an example of:
   a. acute pain.
   b. conscious pain.
   c. chronic pain.
   d. objective pain.

6. Which drug is considered an NSAID?
   a. Acetaminophen
   b. Codeine
   c. Ibuprofen
   d. Meperidine

7. Which statement about children and pain is true?
   a. Children can easily become addicted to opioid analgesics.
   b. Children who are playing are not in pain.
   c. Past pain experiences affect how a child experiences pain.
   d. Children are more likely to have respiratory depression than adults.

8. Respiratory depression is a side effect of:
   a. acetaminophen.
   b. naloxone.
   c. NSAIDs.
   d. opioid analgesics.

9. The drug naloxone (Narcan):
   a. causes respiratory depression at high doses.
   b. is used as an antidote to ibuprofen overdose.
   c. is a topical anesthetic.
   d. is used to reverse the effects of fentanyl.

10. The nurse is preparing an in-service on pain assessment tools for newly graduated nurses who are working in a pediatric department. What information should the nurse include in the teaching?
    a. The FACES scale should be used with children in critical care settings.
    b. The COMFORT scale should be used with preverbal or nonverbal children.
    c. The APPT scale can be used with children as young as 4 years old.
    d. The CRIES scale can be used for neonates and infants younger than 6 months old.

11. The nurse is caring for a 7-year-old who had an appendectomy 2 hours ago. Which pain indicators would the nurse expect to observe? *(Choose all that apply.)*
    a. Strong fear of bodily injury
    b. Thrashing of arms and legs
    c. Bargaining to delay procedure
    d. Denying pain to avoid taking medicine
    e. Understanding cause and effect
    f. Ability to describe intensity of pain

16 The Child with a Fluid and Electrolyte Alteration

HELPFUL HINT

Review the concepts of fluid and electrolyte balance in a biochemistry textbook.

STUDENT LEARNING EXERCISES

Definitions

Match each term with its definition.

1. _____ Acidosis

2. _____ Alkalosis

3. _____ Anuria

4. _____ ECF (extracellular fluid)

5. _____ Hypernatremic (hypertonic) dehydration

6. _____ Hyponatremic (hypotonic) dehydration

7. _____ ICF (intracellular fluid)

8. _____ Interstitial fluid

9. _____ Intravascular fluid

10. _____ Isonatremic (isotonic) dehydration

11. _____ Oliguria

a. Serum pH <7.35
b. Serum sodium >150 mEq/L
c. Serum pH >7.45
d. Fluid found within the cells
e. Absence of urine formation
f. Condition that occurs when solute concentration falls below that of normal body fluids
g. Fluid found outside the cells
h. Fluid surrounding the cells, including lymph fluid
i. Fluid within the blood vessels
j. Diminished amounts of urine output
k. Condition that occurs when solute concentration is identical to that of body fluids

Review of Fluid and Electrolyte Imbalances in Children

Answer as either true (T) or false (F).

12. _____ Sensible water loss is water that is lost through the respiratory tract and skin.

13. _____ Infants' higher rates of peristalsis make them more prone to fluid loss than are older children.

14. _____ Infants' immature renal function increases their ability to concentrate urine.

15. _____ About 60% of the body's water is located in the extracellular compartment in the newborn infant.

16. _____ Infectious diseases, fever, gastroenteritis, and respiratory infections can all result in fluid volume deficit.

Fill in the blanks.

17. Children are more likely to lose _____ fluid when they have a fever.

18. Body fluids are composed of _____ and _____.

19. The primary electrolyte in the ECF is _____; the primary electrolytes in the ICF are

_____ and _____.

20. The normal serum pH ranges from _____ to _____.

21. What three mechanisms operate to keep the serum pH within the normal range?

    a. _____

    b. _____

    c. _____

22. Two buffers that help maintain normal serum pH are _____ and _____.

23. If the serum pH drops below normal, the rate and depth of respirations will _____.

24. The kidneys help maintain normal serum pH by regulating _____ and _____
    in the blood.

Match each disorder with its clinical manifestations.

25. _____ Hyponatremia

26. _____ Hypernatremia

27. _____ Hypokalemia

28. _____ Hyperkalemia

29. _____ Hypocalcemia

30. _____ Hypercalcemia

a. Muscle weakness, leg cramps, ileus
b. Abdominal cramping, tachycardia, and cold, clammy skin
c. Tetany, positive Chvostek sign, hypotension
d. Itching, weakness, bradycardia
e. Flaccid paralysis, cardiac and respiratory arrest
f. Thirst, peripheral edema, seizures

Match each condition with its causes.

31. _____ Metabolic acidosis

32. _____ Metabolic alkalosis

33. _____ Respiratory acidosis

34. _____ Respiratory alkalosis

a. Ketosis, tissue hypoxia, bicarbonate loss
b. Hyperventilation, sepsis, compensation for metabolic acidosis
c. Airway obstruction, respiratory failure
d. Volume depletion, increased alkali intake

Chapter **16** **The Child with a Fluid and Electrolyte Alteration**

Dehydration

Answer as either true (T) or false (F).

35. _____ Isotonic dehydration occurs when water and electrolytes are lost in the same proportion as they occur in the body.

36. _____ In dehydration, fluid loss occurs first in the intracellular fluid.

37. _____ An infant who has lost 7% of his body weight has moderate dehydration.

38. _____ Treatment for severe diarrhea is aimed at treating or preventing hypovolemic shock.

39. _____ When a child is severely dehydrated, electrolytes such as potassium are replaced by administering them by slow IV push.

40. _____ Either lactated Ringer's solution or 0.9% sodium chloride solution is the fluid of choice for parenteral rehydration.

41. _____ Diluted Gatorade or another sports drink is an acceptable oral rehydrating solution for a toddler.

Diarrhea

42. Define diarrhea. _____

_____

43. Diarrhea caused by infection is usually called _____.

44. List four other causes of diarrhea.

    a. _____.

    b. _____

    c. _____

    d. _____

45. Why are sports drinks such as Gatorade inappropriate fluid choices for children with diarrhea?

_____

_____

46. Explain why an infant with diarrhea should continue to receive breast milk or full-strength formula.

_____

_____

47. What common foods are generally well tolerated during diarrhea? _____

_____

100

48. How can skin breakdown be prevented in infants with diarrhea? _____

_____

Vomiting

Answer as either true (T) or false (F).

49. _____ Vomiting can result from allergic reactions.

50. _____ Emesis with a fecal odor may indicate lower intestinal obstruction.

51. _____ Projectile vomiting is usually the result of overfeeding.

52. _____ Oral rehydrating solutions should not be used when a child is vomiting.

53. _____ An infant who has been vomiting should be positioned side-lying or upright to prevent aspiration.

SUGGESTED LEARNING ACTIVITIES

1. Design an information sheet describing dehydration for new parents. Be sure to include the following information about dehydration: what causes it, what to look for, what to do if it occurs, and when to call the physician. Make your information sheet attractive, accurate, and concise.

2. Compare the ingredients in Pedialyte with those in Gatorade. How are they alike? How are they different?

STUDENT LEARNING APPLICATIONS

Enhance your learning by discussing your answers with other students.

Two-month-old Nathan is admitted to the hospital with severe dehydration.

1. As Nathan's nurse, what would you expect to find when assessing the following?

    a. Skin turgor _____

    b. Pulse _____

    c. Urine output _____

    d. Blood pressure _____

    e. Anterior fontanel _____

    f. Sensorium _____

    g. Mucous membranes _____

    h. Skin color _____

2. Because Nathan is not drinking, the physician orders IV fluids. Nathan currently weighs 9 pounds, 4 ounces. What are his 24-hour fluid maintenance requirements?

3. Nathan has not voided for at least 4 hours. The physician has included potassium chloride in the IV order. What problem does this pose? How would you handle it?

4. How will you recognize when Nathan is improving?

Chapter **16** **The Child with a Fluid and Electrolyte Alteration**

Choose the best answer.

1. An otherwise healthy infant is admitted to the hospital with dehydration and diarrhea. She is hyperirritable and agitated. She has flushed skin and dry mucous membranes. The nurse suspects:
   a. hypercalcemia.
   b. hypokalemia.
   c. hyperkalemia.
   d. hypernatremia.

2. An infant who has been vomiting frequently is at risk for:
   a. metabolic acidosis.
   b. metabolic alkalosis.
   c. respiratory acidosis.
   d. respiratory alkalosis.

3. Which statement about the compensatory mechanisms that maintain normal serum pH is true?
   a. If serum pH rises above normal, the respiratory rate and depth increase.
   b. If serum pH rises above normal, the kidneys conserve hydrogen ions.
   c. Bicarbonate is a chemical that buffers the intracellular fluid.
   d. Respiratory compensatory mechanisms work more slowly than renal mechanisms.

4. What are indicators of dehydration in a 4-year-old child?
   a. Heart rate of 120 beats per minute and sunken fontanel
   b. Specific gravity of 1.010 and oliguria
   c. Weight gain and absence of tears
   d. Thirst and specific gravity of 1.038

5. Infants with dehydration must be monitored for signs of impending shock. What is a late sign of shock in the infant?
   a. Decreased blood pressure
   b. Elevated heart rate
   c. Change in skin color
   d. Change in sensorium

6. A preschooler with moderate diarrhea who has just been admitted to the hospital and who is not NPO wants something to drink. The nurse's best choice is to offer:
   a. an oral rehydrating solution.
   b. bottled water.
   c. diluted apple juice.
   d. low-fat milk.

7. An infant with diarrhea has tolerated clear liquids but begins having diarrhea again when she returns to her regular formula. Her diet should be changed to:
   a. boiled skim milk.
   b. soy formula.
   c. IV fluids.
   d. Pedialyte.

8. A child weighing 14 kg is receiving maintenance IV fluids. The child should receive how many milliliters per hour?
   a. 14
   b. 24
   c. 50
   d. 100

9. An infant weighed 6.4 kg at the pediatrician's office 2 days ago. He has had diarrhea since then and he now weighs 5.9 kg. His mucous membranes are dry, his fontanel is sunken, and his capillary refill is about 5 seconds. His serum sodium level is 140 mEq/L. The infant has:
   a. hypotonic dehydration.
   b. moderate dehydration.
   c. hypernatremic dehydration.
   d. severe dehydration.

10. An infant has viral gastroenteritis. To prevent its spread to other family members, the nurse teaches the family:
    a. proper hand hygiene techniques.
    b. how to administer antidiarrheal medications.
    c. how to administer antibiotics.
    d. how to calculate daily fluid requirements.

11. The nurse is teaching a group of new pediatric nurses how to administer potassium in pediatric patients. Which statement made by one of the nurses would indicate a correct understanding of the teaching?
    a. "I should slowly push potassium chloride though a peripheral intravenous line."
    b. "I can administer potassium chloride if the urinary output is less than 1 mL/kg/hr."
    c. "I should add potassium chloride with the IV bag laying flat."
    d. "I can administer potassium chloride at a rate of 1 mEq/kg/hr."

12. The nurse is caring for a 6-year-old with hyponatremic dehydration. Which clinical manifestation(s) should the nurse expect to observe? *(Choose all that apply.)*
    a. Decreased urinary output
    b. Fair skin turgor
    c. Excessive thirst
    d. Dry mucous membranes
    e. Cold skin temperature
    f. Extreme lethargy

13. The nurse is teaching a parent about caring for a 6-month-old with mild diarrhea at home. Which statement made by the parent would indicate a need for additional teaching?
    a. "I should continue to breastfeed my infant and give Pedialyte to supplement even if the diarrhea continues."
    b. "I should wash my hands after I change my infant's diaper and disinfect the diaper changing table frequently."
    c. "I should contact my primary health care provider if my infant does not have a wet diaper after 12 hours."
    d. "I should use mild soap and water instead of diaper wipes to clean my infant after each bowel movement."

Chapter **16** **The Child with a Fluid and Electrolyte Alteration**

17 The Child with an Infectious Disease

HELPFUL HINT

Review the concept of immunity in an anatomy and physiology textbook. Review specific vaccines and immunization schedules in a pharmacology textbook.

STUDENT LEARNING EXERCISES

Definitions

Match each term with its definition.

1. _____ Exanthem
2. _____ Host
3. _____ Immunity
4. _____ Infection
5. _____ Pathogen
6. _____ Prodrome
7. _____ Toxin
8. _____ Vector

a. Invasion of an organism by another organism
b. Microorganism that produces disease
c. An eruption or rash on the skin
d. A carrier that transfers an infective agent from one host to another
e. Initial stage of a disease
f. Poison produced by pathogenic microorganisms
g. Resistance of the body to the effects of harmful organisms
h. Organism from which a parasite obtains its nourishment

Transmission of Pathogens

Match each mode of infection transmission with its description.

9. _____ Airborne route
10. _____ Fecal-oral transmission
11. _____ Direct contact transmission
12. _____ Vector borne
13. _____ Direct inoculation

a. Infection contracted through the use of contaminated needles
b. Transmission of disease through sexual activity
c. Illness resulting from a deer tick bite
d. Infection caused by pathogens shed through sneezing or coughing
e. Illness caused by ingestion of contaminated food

Infection and Host Defenses

14. The first lines of defense in an intact immune system are the _____ and _____.

Viral Infections

Match each virus with its description.

15. _____ Cytomegalovirus (CMV)

16. _____ Epstein-Barr virus

17. _____ Fifth disease

18. _____ Mumps

19. _____ Poliomyelitis

20. _____ Rabies

21. _____ Roseola infantum

22. _____ Rubella

23. _____ Rubeola

24. _____ Varicella zoster

25. _____ Variola

a. Infection may proceed to paralysis
b. Most cases occur between 6 and 18 months of age
c. Acute signs of fever, pharyngitis, lymphadenopathy, and hepatosplenomegaly continue for 2 to 4 weeks, followed by gradual recovery
d. Virus remains latent in a sensory nerve ending and the dorsal root ganglion and may be reactivated later
e. Its vaccine can be given after exposure to the virus
f. This is a common cause of congenital infections in infants
g. Koplik spots in the buccal mucosa appear 2 days before the red, maculopapular rash
h. Its classic sign is parotid glandular swelling
i. This is a mild systemic disease with a fiery red edematous facial rash followed by a maculopapular rash on the trunk and extremities
j. Infection during the first trimester of pregnancy has serious consequences for the fetus
k. Immunization after exposure provides protection against a fatal outcome

26. Describe three interventions to relieve discomfort from skin irritation caused by a viral exanthem.

a. _____

b. _____

c. _____

Bacterial, Rickettsial, Borrelia, Helminth, and Fungal Infections

Answer as either true (T) or false (F).

27. _____ Pertussis is a highly contagious disease associated with a high mortality rate.

28. _____ Scarlet fever is caused by group A beta-hemolytic streptococci.

29. _____ In both Lyme disease and Rocky Mountain spotted fever, the vector is a tick.

30. _____ When a child is diagnosed with a helminthic infection, treatment is usually provided for the entire family.

31. _____ Frequent hand hygiene can prevent the spread of parasitic infections.

32. _____ Manifestations of fungal infections appear rapidly after the child is exposed to the organism.

33. _____ The organisms that most frequently cause neonatal sepsis are *Escherichia coli* and group B *Streptococcus*.

34. _____ The early signs of neonatal sepsis may be vague and nonspecific.

35. _____ A bull's-eye rash may be a manifestation of diphtheria.

36. _____ An opportunistic fungal infection is limited to the skin, hair, and nails.

37. _____ Children should receive a pertussis booster (Tdap) between the ages of 11 and 12.

Sexually Transmissible Infections (STIs)

38. How has *ophthalmia neonatorum* been controlled? _____

_____.

39. Children who acquire STIs after the neonatal period should be evaluated for what?

_____

40. The classic signs of congenital syphilis include _____,

_____ and _____.

41. How do infants become infected with *Chlamydia?* _____

_____

42. Name the three ways in which gonorrhea can be transmitted.

a. _____

b. _____

c. _____

Match each disease with its treatment.

43. _____ Gonorrhea

44. _____ Syphilis

45. _____ Chlamydia

46. _____ Trichomoniasis

47. _____ Human papillomavirus

48. _____ Bacterial vaginosis

49. _____ Herpes simplex virus 2

a. Metronidazole
b. Erythromycin
c. Clindamycin
d. Ceftriaxone
e. Acyclovir
f. Penicillin
g. Surgery

SUGGESTED LEARNING ACTIVITIES

1. Plan a 30-minute presentation on the importance of immunizations for a parents' meeting at a day care center. What information is essential to include? How would you convey the importance of immunizations? How would you evaluate the effectiveness of your presentation?

2. Obtain information from the local health department on sexually transmissible infections. Plan a presentation for adolescents on how to prevent STIs with the information you gathered.

106

STUDENT LEARNING APPLICATIONS

Enhance your learning by discussing your answers with other students.

Seven-year-old Jodie has been admitted to the hospital for oxygen therapy and IV antibiotics for the treatment of pneumonia. Ten days ago, her best friend came down with chickenpox. Jodie has never had chickenpox and has not yet received the varicella vaccine.

1. Does Jodie require isolation? Why or why not?

Two days after admission, Jodie develops a macular rash on her trunk and scalp, and her fever returns.

2. How will this alter the isolation procedure?

3. Will she be given acyclovir? Why or why not?

4. Will she be given varicella zoster immune globulin? Why or why not?

When entering Jodie's room to take vital signs, the nurse finds her crying. She refuses to eat her lunch, saying she wants to go to the playroom.

5. How should the nurse handle this situation?

Jodie is uncomfortable from the itching caused by the skin lesions. You find her scratching her arms and trunk.

6. What interventions would you implement to relieve the itching and prevent scratching?

REVIEW QUESTIONS

Choose the best answer.

1. Congenital rubella infection may result in:
   a. encephalitis.
   b. cardiac anomalies.
   c. hydronephrosis.
   d. neural tube defects.

2. Splenic rupture is a complication of:
   a. CMV infection.
   b. Epstein-Barr virus.
   c. erythema infectiosum.
   d. varicella zoster.

3. Which nursing intervention is not appropriate when caring for a child with pertussis?
   a. Monitoring intake and output.
   b. Maintaining enteric precautions.
   c. Providing child with periods of uninterrupted rest.
   d. Administering erythromycin as ordered.

4. A "white strawberry tongue" is a clinical manifestation of which infectious disease?
   a. Poliomyelitis
   b. Roseola
   c. Rubeola
   d. Scarlet fever

5. Using an insect repellent when in the woods can help prevent:
   a. CMV infection.
   b. helminth infections.
   c. Rocky Mountain spotted fever.
   d. scarlet fever.

6. Which of these statements about sexually transmissible infections (STIs) is false?
   a. Sexual abuse is suspected when a toddler or preschooler has a gonorrheal infection.
   b. Syphilis can be transmitted from mother to fetus through the placenta.
   c. Males with trichomoniasis usually have a urethral discharge and dysuria.
   d. Chronic respiratory problems are a complication of a neonatal chlamydial infection.

7. An adolescent comes to the clinic because she has dysuria, urinary frequency, and a mucopurulent discharge. These signs are manifestations of which sexually transmissible infection?
   a. Herpes simplex virus
   b. Bacterial vaginosis
   c. Chlamydia
   d. Human papillomavirus

8. Which description matches the rash associated with Lyme disease?
   a. Erythematous maculopapular rash surrounded by a whitish ring
   b. Fine, red papular rash that appears within 24 hours of tick bite
   c. Petechial rash that begins on extremities and spreads to the rest of the body
   d. Erythematous macula or papule with a clearing in the center

9. The nurse is caring for a 7-year-old with viral exanthema. Which intervention(s) should the nurse include in the child's plan of care? *(Choose all that apply.)*
   a. Provide comfort with soothing lotions.
   b. Restrict activity to quiet activities.
   c. Administer appropriate dose of baby aspirin for a fever.
   d. Provide warm humidification for a cough.
   e. Encourage frequent drinking of cool liquids.

10. The nurse is teaching the parent of a 15-year-old with infectious mononucleosis. Which statement made by the parent would indicate an understanding of the teaching?
    a. "I should expect my child to return to normal activities within 5 days."
    b. "I should offer my child soothing liquids and bland foods for a sore throat."
    c. "I can administer aspirin to my child for a fever higher than 100° F."
    d. "I can allow my child to actively play with siblings as long as they stay in the house."

11. The nurse is talking to a group of adolescents about sexually transmissible infections (STIs). What information should the nurse include? *(Choose all that apply.)*
    a. All STIs have some type of rash as the first sign of an infection.
    b. Many STIs can be cured by completing a course of antibiotics.
    c. Some STIs can cause sterility, cancer, and death.
    d. STIs are transmitted only through sexual intercourse.
    e. Many STIs cannot be cured but have treatments to relieve the symptoms.
    f. STIs can be eliminated with the use of a male or female condom.

18 The Child with an Immunologic Alteration

HELPFUL HINT

Review the immune system in an anatomy and physiology textbook.

STUDENT LEARNING EXERCISES

Definitions

Match each term with its definition.

1. _____ Active immunity

2. _____ Allergy

3. _____ Antibody

4. _____ Antigen

5. _____ Autoimmune disease

6. _____ Complement

7. _____ Immune system

8. _____ Immunodeficiency

9. _____ Leukocytes

10. _____ Lymphocytes

11. _____ Nonspecific immune functions

12. _____ Passive immunity

13. _____ Specific immune functions

a. Blood cells that mainly function to protect the body against foreign substances
b. Production of autoantibodies against cells of the body by the immune system
c. Protection occurring when serum containing an antibody is given to someone without the antibody
d. Protection that follows exposure to an antigen
e. A defect in the immune system that places a person at high risk for infection
f. Hypersensitivity reaction
g. Primary white blood cells of the immune system
h. Body's internal defense against foreign substances
i. Substance identified by the immune system as foreign
j. Protein produced by the immune system that binds to specific antigens and eliminates them from the body
k. Accessory system to a humoral response composed of proteins that facilitate enzyme action and antigen death
l. Humoral and cell-mediated responses that are activated in a highly discriminatory manner
m. Protective barriers that are activated in the presence of an antigen but are not specific to that antigen

Review of the Immune System

Match the cells with their functions.

14. _____ Neutrophils

15. _____ Eosinophils

16. _____ Basophils

17. _____ Monocytes

18. _____ B lymphocytes

19. _____ T lymphocytes

a. Kill target cells directly
b. Responsible for cellular immunity
c. The first leukocytes to respond to tissue damage
d. Ingest and introduce antigens into the circulation
e. Inhibit the actions of helper T and B cells
f. Neutralize histamine
g. Responsible for humoral immunity
h. Secrete lymphokines that stimulate B cells to manufacture antibodies
i. Secrete histamine, heparin, and serotonin in inflammatory and hypersensitivity reactions

109

20. _____ Helper (CD4+) T cells

21. _____ Suppressor T cells

22. _____ Cytotoxic (CD8+) T cells

Answer as either true (T) or false (F).

23. _____ The production of antibodies signals the beginning of the nonspecific immune response.

24. _____ The immune complexes include the bone marrow, thymus, spleen, lymph nodes, and tissue.

25. _____ Antibodies are also called immunoglobulins.

26. _____ Transfer of maternal antibodies to the fetus through the placenta is an example of active immunity.

Human Immunodeficiency Virus (HIV) Infection

27. Name three ways HIV infection can be transmitted from mother to child.

a. _____

b. _____

c. _____

28. The rate of HIV transmission from mother to child decreases when both receive _____.

29. Describe *PCP prophylaxis* for an infant exposed to HIV. _____

_____

_____

30. The dosage of antiretroviral combination drug therapy for an adolescent is based on what?

_____

Corticosteroid Therapy

31. How do corticosteroids cause immunosuppression? _____

_____

_____

32. Why is it dangerous to abruptly stop corticosteroid medication? _____

_____

33. Corticosteroid excess is diagnosed by administering a bolus of _____.

34. If long-term use of corticosteroids is required, they are usually prescribed to be taken _____

_____

35. For a child receiving corticosteroids, what can be done to minimize the risk for gastrointestinal bleeding?

_____

_____

To deal with increased appetite? _____

_____

Immune Complex and Autoimmune Disorders

36. Give two examples of immune complex disorders.

a. _____

b. _____

37. What are autoantibodies? _____

_____

Systemic Lupus Erythematosus (SLE)

Answer as either true (T) or false (F).

38. _____ SLE has periods of remission and exacerbation.

39. _____ SLE affects more males than females.

40. _____ In SLE, antinuclear antibodies are present.

41. _____ In SLE, systemic corticosteroids are used to control inflammation.

42. _____ The clinical manifestations of SLE depend on which body systems are affected.

43. _____ Antimalarial drugs are used to treat renal disorders in SLE.

Allergic Reactions and Anaphylaxis

44. What is an allergy? _____

_____

Match each allergic reaction with its example.

45. _____ Immediate hypersensitivity

46. _____ Cytotoxic hypersensitivity

47. _____ Arthus hypersensitivity

48. _____ Delayed cell-mediated hypersensitivity

a. Transfusion reaction
b. Asthma
c. Poison ivy
d. Poststreptococcal glomerulonephritis

49. List the most serious features of anaphylaxis. _____

_____

Chapter **18** **The Child with an Immunologic Alteration**

50. What is an *Epi-Pen?* _____

_____

51. What are the differences between allergy skin tests and the RAST test? _____

_____

_____

STUDENT LEARNING ACTIVITY

Many communities have support groups for people with SLE. Attend a meeting and then report about the meeting to your class.

STUDENT LEARNING APPLICATIONS

Enhance your learning by discussing your answers with other students.

Caring for a child with HIV infection or AIDS can be very challenging from both the physical and psychologic perspectives. It is important for health care professionals to be aware of their own feelings about the disease. Think about the following questions and then discuss them with a family member, friend, or another student.

1. Which aspects of caring for a child with HIV or AIDS would you personally find most difficult?

    a. Providing physical care: _____

    b. Worrying about contracting HIV from the child: _____

    c. Dealing with the child's family: _____

    d. Knowing that the child has a life-threatening illness: _____

    e. Meeting the child's psychosocial needs: _____

2. If the child contracted HIV prenatally, how would you feel about the child's mother? Could you remain nonjudgmental and supportive?

3. Which HIV-positive adolescent would be most difficult for you to care for? Which one would be the least difficult? Why?
    a. 14-year-old Annie, who uses illegal IV drugs
    b. 16-year-old Beth, who is a teenage prostitute
    c. 17-year-old David, who is homosexual

REVIEW QUESTIONS

Choose the best answer.

1. When the immune system fails to differentiate the body's cells from foreign cells, what occurs?
    a. Active immunity
    b. Autoimmune response
    c. Cell-mediated response
    d. Humoral response

2. IgA:
    a. crosses the placenta.
    b. provides antibacterial protection.
    c. passes to the neonate through breast milk.
    d. influences B-cell differentiation.

3. The test used to assess the immune status of an HIV-positive child is:
    a. CD4+ count.
    b. ELISA.
    c. HIV culture.
    d. p24 antigen.

4. The nurse is teaching a parent about corticosteroid treatment. Which statement made by the parent would indicate the need for additional teaching?
    a. "I should have my child take the medication with food or milk."
    b. "I should avoid stopping the medication abruptly."
    c. "I can expect the drug to mask usual signs of infection."
    d. "I can expect to see changes in physical appearance that are permanent but minor."

5. Which symptom(s) would the nurse expect to observe in a 16-year-old with systemic lupus erythematosus? *(Choose all that apply.)*
    a. Erythema marginatum and chorea
    b. Discoid rash and photosensitivity
    c. Fever and erythematous rash
    d. Laryngospasm and edema
    e. Painless lesions and swollen joints

6. The antibody involved in allergic reactions is:
    a. IgA.
    b. IgD.
    c. IgE.
    d. IgG.

7. Most children with HIV are infected:
    a. through blood and blood products.
    b. perinatally.
    c. through sexual abuse.
    d. through failure to use Standard Precautions.

8. Prophylaxis for *Pneumocystis jiroveci* includes:
    a. trimethoprim-sulfamethoxazole.
    b. corticosteroids.
    c. immunoglobulins.
    d. all of the above.

9. The school nurse is discussing an upcoming field trip to the zoo with two sixth graders who are allergic to bees. Which statement made by one of the students indicates that he or she needs further clarification about their condition?
    a. "I'll make sure that I wear khakis instead of jeans that day."
    b. "When bees come near me, I will run away as fast as I can."
    c. "If I have to use my Epi-Pen, I can inject it right into my thigh without pulling my khakis down."
    d. "I'll keep the windows closed in the bus."

10. The nurse is teaching the parent of an 11-year-old about the administration of prednisone (Prednisolone). Which statement made by the parent would indicate a correct understanding of the teaching?
a. "I should give the prednisone to my child with milk."
b. "I should store the prednisone in a warm area of the kitchen."
c. "I can expect my child to have a low-grade fever and fatigue while taking prednisone."
d. "I can allow my child to take a nonsteroidal antiinflammatory drug for muscle pain while taking prednisone."

11. The nurse is preparing an in-service about highly indicative clinical manifestations of immunodeficiency in children for a group of new pediatric nurses. Which topic(s) should the nurse include in the in-service teaching? *(Choose all that apply.)*
a. Persistent respiratory infections
b. Persistent thrush
c. Failure to thrive
d. Repeated otitis media
e. Poor response to therapy
f. Hepatosplenomegaly

19 The Child with a Gastrointestinal Alteration

HELPFUL HINT

Review the anatomy and physiology of the gastrointestinal tract in an anatomy and physiology textbook.

STUDENT LEARNING EXERCISES

Definitions

Match each term with its definition.

1. _____ Achalasia
2. _____ Atresia
3. _____ Azotemia
4. _____ Dysphagia
5. _____ Encopresis
6. _____ Fistula
7. _____ Fundoplication
8. _____ Hematemesis
9. _____ Melena
10. _____ Occult bleeding
11. _____ Peristalsis
12. _____ Projectile vomiting
13. _____ Pylorus
14. _____ Tenesmus

a. Presence of urea in the blood
b. Distal opening of the stomach
c. Black, tarry stools, indicating bleeding
d. Abnormal passage between two organs
e. Progressive wavelike motions that propel fluid and food through gastrointestinal tract
f. Failure of smooth muscle fibers of the gastrointestinal tract to relax
g. Incontinence of feces
h. Surgical wrapping of the stomach fundus around distal esophagus to prevent gastric reflux
i. Forceful vomiting
j. Abnormal closure or absence of a body passage or orifice
k. Vomiting of blood, either red or "coffee grounds"
l. Inability to swallow or difficulty in swallowing
m. Bleeding that is detectable only by microscopic or chemical means
n. Ineffective, painful, or continuous urge to defecate

Review of the Gastrointestinal System

15. What are the primary functions of the upper gastrointestinal system? _____

_____

16. What are the primary functions of the lower gastrointestinal system? _____

_____

17. What are the functions of the liver? _____

_____

18. Prenatally, how are nutrients brought to and waste products removed from the fetus?

_____

Disorders of Prenatal Development

Answer as either true (T) or false (F).

19. _____ The diagnosis of cleft lip and palate can be determined through inspection.

20. _____ Infants with cleft lip are at risk for problems with parent-infant attachment.

21. _____ Cleft palate repair precedes cleft lip repair.

22. _____ To keep a cleft palate repair incision site clean, the nurse gives water after all feedings.

23. _____ Children with cleft palates require frequent hearing tests.

Fill in the blanks.

24. _____ is a significant prenatal clue in the diagnosis of tracheoesophageal fistula (TEF).

25. An infant with TEF is at constant risk for _____.

26. What are the "3 Cs" that suggest TEF? _____

_____

27. How does an infant with TEF receive nutrition before surgery? _____

_____

28. Describe how to care for an esophagostomy. _____

_____

Match each disorder with its description.

29. _____ Hiatal hernia

30. _____ Congenital diaphragmatic hernia

31. _____ Imperforate anus

32. _____ Gastroschisis

33. _____ Omphalocele

34. _____ Umbilical hernia

a. Condition in which viscera are outside the abdominal cavity and not covered with a sac
b. Incomplete development of the anus
c. Protrusion of a portion of the stomach through the esophageal hiatus of the diaphragm
d. Herniation of the gut into the umbilical cord
e. Herniation of abdominal contents into the thoracic cavity through the diaphragm
f. Condition in which gut pushes outward at the umbilicus during straining or crying

Motility Disorders

35. Describe the home dietary management of gastroesophageal reflux (GER) in a 5-month-old.

_____

_____

36. List the drugs used to treat GER that have the following actions.

   a. Decrease acid secretions: _____

   b. Accelerate gastric emptying: _____

   c. Offer barrier protection: _____

   d. Suppress gastric acid secretion: _____

37. Describe how chronic constipation can lead to encopresis. _____

   _____

38. _____ is thought to be a common cause of irritable bowel syndrome.

39. Clinical manifestations of irritable bowel syndrome include: _____

   _____

Inflammatory and Infectious Diseases

Answer as either true (T) or false (F).

40. _____ Stress ulcers are considered primary ulcers.

41. _____ Dietary management of ulcers includes a bland diet with added milk.

42. _____ *Helicobacter pylori* is a bacterium associated with duodenal ulcers.

43. _____ *Giardia* is the most common pathogen causing gastroenteritis in day care settings.

44. _____ Antimicrobials are used to treat infections caused by rotavirus.

45. _____ In gastroenteritis, dehydration and electrolyte imbalances must be corrected promptly.

46. _____ Headache, irritability, nuchal rigidity, and seizures are manifestations of *Salmonella* infection.

47. _____ The cardinal symptom of appendicitis is pain that eventually localizes at McBurney's point.

48. _____ Sudden cessation of pain in a child with appendicitis is indicative of spontaneous remission.

49. Describe the differences between Crohn's disease and ulcerative colitis. _____

   _____

   _____

   _____

50. Which four categories of drugs are used to treat irritable bowel disease?

   a. _____

   b. _____

Chapter **19** **The Child with a Gastrointestinal Alteration**

c. _____

d. _____

Obstructive Disorders

51. Describe the vomiting that occurs with pyloric stenosis. _____

_____

52. The classic signs of intussusception include _____

_____.

53. How is hydrostatic reduction of an intussusception attempted? _____

54. _____ is caused by a malrotation of the bowel.

55. What is the cardinal sign of Hirschsprung disease in the newborn infant? _____

_____

56. A life-threatening complication of Hirschsprung disease is _____.

Malabsorption Disorders

Answer as either true (T) or false (F).

57. _____ Isomil is an appropriate formula for an infant with lactose intolerance.

58. _____ Celiac disease results from the inability to digest celiac.

59. _____ Corn and rice products must be avoided in celiac disease.

60. _____ Corticosteroids are used to decrease mucosal inflammation in celiac disease.

Hepatic Disorders

For each type of hepatitis, list its mode(s) of transmission.

61. Hepatitis A (HAV): _____

62. Hepatitis B (HBV): _____

63. Hepatitis C (HCV): _____

64. Hepatitis delta (HDV): _____

65. Hepatitis E (HEV): _____

66. List the clinical manifestations for each of the following:

a. *Anicteric phase of acute hepatitis:* _____

_____

b. *Icteric phase of acute hepatitis:* _____

_____

c. *Fulminating hepatitis:* _____

_____

67. Vaccinations are currently available for which forms of hepatitis? _____

_____

Answer as either true (T) or false (F).

68. _____ The hepatitis B vaccine protects against both HBV and HDV.

69. _____ The available hepatitis vaccines are recommended for all infants and children who are not immunocompromised.

70. _____ Hepatitis C is the major indication for liver transplantation in children.

71. _____ The Kasai procedure corrects biliary atresia.

72. _____ In biliary atresia, fat-soluble vitamins are not absorbed.

73. _____ Pruritus can be alleviated with colloidal oatmeal baths.

74. _____ Manifestations of portal hypertension include ascites, gastrointestinal bleeding, and splenomegaly.

Fill in the blanks.

75. The three major complications of cirrhosis are _____

_____

76. _____ is the definitive therapy for cirrhosis.

SUGGESTED LEARNING ACTIVITIES

1. Role play with another student. In this scenario, one of you is the nurse and the other is the parent of a newborn infant with a cleft lip and palate. The parent refuses to hold or even look at the infant. How would the nurse promote parent-infant attachment in this situation? You may want to include another student as an observer or coach.

2. Observe one of the diagnostic procedures discussed in this chapter, such as fiberoptic endoscopy, abdominal flat plate radiographs, or colonoscopy. On the basis of your observations and readings, design a teaching plan for the observed procedure for an 8-year-old.

STUDENT LEARNING APPLICATIONS

Enhance your learning by discussing your answers with other students.

Melissa, a 16 year old, has just been diagnosed with Crohn's disease.

1. From what you know about adolescent development, what would you guess Melissa's chief concerns are about this diagnosis?

Chapter **19** **The Child with a Gastrointestinal Alteration**

2. As her nurse, how would you determine whether your guesses are accurate?

3. How might this disease affect Melissa's physical and psychosocial development?

4. Melissa tells you, "Well, I guess this means that I won't be going to college." How would you respond to this statement?

REVIEW QUESTIONS

Choose the best answer.

1. At his 1-year checkup, you note that Jason has thin arms and legs and abdominal distention. His mother reports that he has been irritable, has lost his appetite, and has foul-smelling stools. He has fallen behind on the growth chart. Jason probably has:
   a. Crohn disease.
   b. Hirschsprung disease.
   c. irritable bowel syndrome.
   d. celiac disease.

2. Which intervention is not appropriate after surgery for Hirschsprung disease?
   a. Assess surgical site for swelling, redness, and drainage.
   b. Monitor rectal temperature every 4 hours for evidence of fever.
   c. Reunite parents with child as soon as possible.
   d. Keep child NPO until bowel sounds return.

3. A 5-year-old who was admitted to rule out appendicitis tells the nurse, "It doesn't hurt anymore." The nurse suspects that the:
   a. child is afraid of surgery.
   b. child has a ruptured appendix.
   c. child wants to please the nurse.
   d. child cannot communicate about pain accurately.

4. A 6-year-old is admitted to the hospital with severe abdominal pain, bloody diarrhea, high fever, headache, and nuchal rigidity. The child probably has:
   a. an intussusception.
   b. cirrhosis.
   c. a perforated appendix.
   d. a *Shigella* infection.

5. For the child with encopresis, mineral oil is often prescribed to:
   a. facilitate absorption of fat-soluble vitamins.
   b. eliminate pain associated with bowel movements.
   c. evacuate fecal impactions.
   d. initiate the normal gastrocolic reflex.

6. An adolescent has just been diagnosed with an ulcer. Which statement indicates that he or she requires clarification about the therapeutic regimen?
   a. "I won't take my ulcer medication and milk of magnesia close together."
   b. "I'll switch to orange soda from cola."
   c. "I'll take two Motrin when the pain comes back."
   d. "I'll stay away from cigarette smoke."

7. When performing a newborn assessment, the nurse observes that the infant is cyanotic and has nasal flaring and retractions. Also, no breath sounds can be auscultated on the left side, and he palpates an apical pulse on the right side of the sternum. The nurse immediately notifies the physician because he suspects:
   a. a tracheoesophageal fistula.
   b. a cleft palate.
   c. pyloric stenosis.
   d. a diaphragmatic hernia.

8. Careful hand hygiene before and after patient contact can prevent the spread of:
   a. hepatitis A.
   b. volvulus.
   c. ulcerative colitis.
   d. all of the above.

9. A child with lactose intolerance may be able to drink milk if it is taken with:
   a. Colace.
   b. Lactaid.
   c. Lactulose (Enulose).
   d. Lomotil (diphenoxylate and atropine).

10. The nurse is teaching the parent of a 2-month-old about the use of elbow restraints after surgical repair of a cleft lip. Which statement made by the parent would indicate a need for additional teaching?
    a. "The restraints may be removed while my infant sleeps."
    b. "The restraints will be removed for 10 to 15 minutes every 2 hours."
    c. "The restraints will be applied loosely but tight enough to prevent elbow bending."
    d. "The restraints will be used for the next 8 days."

11. A newborn with a tracheoesophageal fistula is waiting for transfer to a neonatal intensive care unit. The nurse's priority intervention is:
    a. arranging for transportation.
    b. preventing aspiration.
    c. providing psychosocial support for the parents.
    d. providing small, frequent feedings.

12. Which test is not typically ordered when gastroesophageal reflux is suspected?
    a. Fiberoptic endoscopy
    b. Barium enema
    c. pH studies
    d. Scintigraphy

13. The nurse is teaching a group of pediatric nurses about gastroesophageal reflux disease (GERD). What information should be included in the teaching? *(Choose all that apply.)*
    a. The peak incidence of GERD occurs at 4 months of age.
    b. The common sign of GERD is vomiting after a meal.
    c. The prone position is recommended for infants with GERD.
    d. The feeding pattern for GERD is large feedings, spaced 4 hours apart.
    e. The teaching for parents with an infant with GERD should include CPR.
    f. The use of a pacifier with an infant with GERD is encouraged to reduce crying.

14. Which clinical manifestation(s) would a nurse expect to see in a neonate with a congenital diaphragmatic hernia? *(Choose all that apply.)*
    a. Herniation of gut into umbilical cord
    b. Scaphoid abdomen
    c. Diminished breath sounds on affected side
    d. Increased peristalsis
    e. Nasal flaring and retractions
    f. Coughing and wheezing

Chapter **19** **The Child with a Gastrointestinal Alteration**

15. The nurse is caring for a 12-year-old with suspected appendicitis. Indicate on the picture where McBurney's point is.

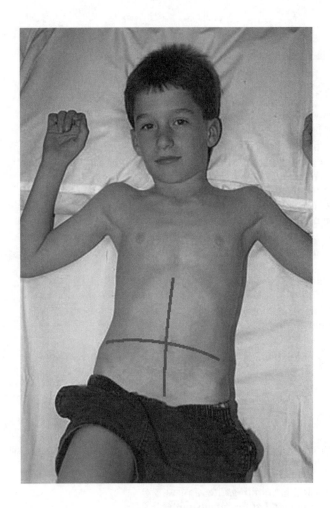

20 The Child with a Genitourinary Alteration

Review the anatomy and physiology of the renal system in an anatomy and physiology textbook.

STUDENT LEARNING EXERCISES

Definitions

Match each term with its definition.

1. _____ Arteriovenous fistula

2. _____ Arteriovenous graft

3. _____ Dysuria

4. _____ Edema

5. _____ Frequency

6. _____ Hypercalciuria

7. _____ Hyperlipidemia

8. _____ Hypoalbuminemia

9. _____ Proteinuria

10. _____ Urgency

a. Sudden urge to urinate
b. Excessive calcium in the urine
c. Presence of protein in the urine
d. Tube inserted between an artery and a vein for hemodialysis
e. Presence of abnormally large amounts of fluid in intercellular spaces of the body
f. Connection between an artery and a vein
g. Low levels of albumin in the blood
h. High levels of serum cholesterol and triglycerides
i. Pain when urinating
j. Urination at short time intervals

Review of the Genitourinary System

11. The newborn infant's bladder is located in the _____ cavity.

12. Children's shorter urethras predispose them to _____.

13. The _____ is the kidney's functional unit.

14. A child's bladder capacity is approximately equal to _____ mL/kg of body weight.

15. Normal urine pH ranges from _____ to _____.

Enuresis

Answer as either true (T) or false (F).

16. _____ Diurnal enuresis may be helped by biofeedback.

17. _____ Imipramine, an antidepressant, may be prescribed for nocturnal enuresis.

18. _____ Secondary enuresis is frequently the result of stress.

Urinary Tract Infections

Match each disorder with its description.

19. _____ Cystitis

20. _____ Pyelonephritis

21. _____ Hydronephrosis

22. _____ Vesicoureteral reflux

a. Structural defect that allows urine to back-flow into the ureters
b. Inflammation of the bladder
c. Kidney infection
d. Dilation of the kidney

Fill in the blanks.

23. The diagnostic study for a urinary tract infection is a _____.

24. Bladder catheterization and _____ are two ways of collecting a urine specimen that will accurately detect bacteria in the urine.

25. A voiding cystourethrogram is ordered to detect _____.

26. Pyelonephritis is treated with _____ antibiotics.

27. Hypertension in childhood might result from renal scarring resulting from _____.

28. List five ways of preventing urinary tract infections in young children.

    a. _____

    b. _____

    c. _____

    d. _____

    e. _____

Cryptorchidism

Answer as either true (T) or false (F).

29. _____ Preterm infants have a higher incidence of cryptorchidism than do term infants.

30. _____ Most infants with cryptorchidism require surgery.

31. _____ Orchiopexy is the surgical correction for cryptorchidism.

32. _____ Children with cryptorchidism are at increased risk for testicular cancer.

Hypospadias and Epispadias

Fill in the blanks.

33. Infants with hypospadias should not be _____ before surgical correction.

34. Dorsal placement of the urethral opening in males is called _____; ventral placement is called _____.

35. _____ is a downward curvature of the penile shaft.

36. After surgical urinary diversions, such as indwelling catheters or _____, are used to allow the meatus to heal.

Miscellaneous Disorders and Anomalies of the Genitourinary Tract

Match each disorder with its description.

37. _____ Hydrocele

38. _____ Phimosis

39. _____ Testicular torsion

40. _____ Bladder exstrophy

41. _____ Ovotesticular disorder of sex development (DSD)

a. Inability to retract the prepuce after about 3 years of age
b. Presence of both ovarian and testicular tissues
c. Painless swelling of the scrotum
d. Urinary bladder located outside of the body at birth
e. Painful swelling of the scrotum

Acute Poststreptococcal Glomerulonephritis

42. List the clinical manifestations of acute poststreptococcal glomerulonephritis. _____

_____

_____

43. Describe the role that antigen-antibody complexes play in acute poststreptococcal glomerulonephritis.

_____

_____

44. In severe renal insufficiency, blood urea nitrogen and serum creatinine _____.

45. _____ indicates that acute poststreptococcal glomerulonephritis is starting to resolve.

Nephrotic Syndrome

46. List the clinical manifestations of nephrotic syndrome. _____

_____

_____

47. Which drug is used initially to achieve remission in nephrotic syndrome? _____

_____

48. When is nephrotic syndrome considered to be in remission? _____

_____

Acute Renal Failure

Match each disorder with the type of acute renal failure it causes. (Answers may be used more than once.)

49. _____ Glomerulonephritis

50. _____ Pyelonephritis

51. _____ Dehydration

52. _____ Hemolytic uremic syndrome

53. _____ Hemorrhagic shock

54. _____ Neurogenic bladder

55. _____ Vesicoureteral reflux

a. Prerenal
b. Intrarenal
c. Postrenal

Answer as either true (T) or false (F).

56. _____ Hemolytic uremic syndrome is the most frequent cause of acute renal failure in children.

57. _____ Kayexalate is administered to manage hypokalemia.

58. _____ Hyponatremia results from fluid overload in acute renal failure.

59. _____ Metabolic alkalosis develops in acute renal failure in children.

Chronic Renal Failure and End-Stage Renal Disease

60. Dialysis removes _____ and _____ from the blood and

    regulates _____ and _____.

61. Vascular access for hemodialysis is achieved through a double-lumen central line or a(n) _____

    _____.

62. In peritoneal dialysis, the dialysis fluid is placed in the _____ cavity.

63. Manifestations of end-stage renal disease include _____

    _____.

64. Children with ESRD require either dialysis or _____.

65. _____ is the most common complication of kidney transplantation.

66. Children with kidney transplants are at high risk for infection because of _____

    _____.

SUGGESTED LEARNING ACTIVITIES

1. Visit a dialysis center and interview one of the nurses. Describe to your class what you thought was the most challenging aspects of the nurse's work.

2. Contact a medical supply company. Find out the cost of the equipment and supplies needed for peritoneal dialysis. Calculate the approximate cost per month. Find out whether the costs are covered entirely by medical insurance. Report your findings to your class.

STUDENT LEARNING APPLICATIONS

Enhance your learning by discussing your answers with other students.

Five-year-old Jack is brought to the pediatrician by his parents, who noticed that Jack has puffiness around his eyes and ankles and that his belly seems to be getting bigger. They also report that he doesn't seem like himself and that he has no appetite. You find that his vital signs are within normal limits for his age and sex. You note pitting edema of his lower extremities and abdomen. Urine tests are negative for occult blood and +4 for protein.

1. On the basis of these findings, what would you expect Jack's diagnosis to be?

    After a brief hospitalization, Jack is discharged and sent home. His symptoms should be treated with prednisone and penicillin; he is on a no-added-salt diet.

2. What will you tell the family about the actions and side effects of prednisone and how to administer it?

3. Because the physician told Jack's mother that he doesn't have an infection, she does not understand the need for penicillin. How will you explain the reason for the drug?

4. How will you explain the need for the no-added-salt diet?

REVIEW QUESTIONS

Choose the best answer.

1. A 7-year-old with cystitis will require:
    a. a renal ultrasound.
    b. oral antibiotics.
    c. a suprapubic aspiration.
    d. all of the above.

2. Which observations and prior history should the nurse expect when caring for a 9-year-old with a suspected diagnosis of acute poststreptococcal glomerulonephritis? *(Choose all that apply.)*
    a. Back pain for the past 2 days
    b. Tea-colored urine
    c. A history of hypertension
    d. A sore throat 10 days ago
    e. Periorbital edema
    f. Acute abdominal pain

3. A child with nephrotic syndrome who is steroid dependent:
    a. will be put on an alternate-day dosing schedule of steroids.
    b. initially responds well to prednisone but relapses while on a tapering schedule.
    c. continues to have proteinuria after 8 weeks of steroid therapy.
    d. will eventually require dialysis.

4. A child with grade 1 vesicoureteral reflux is treated with:
    a. antibiotics.
    b. diuretics.
    c. muscle relaxants.
    d. surgery.

5. Recurrent urinary tract infections are clinical manifestations of:
    a. enuresis.
    b. hypospadias.
    c. glomerulonephritis.
    d. vesicoureteral reflux.

127

6. A 5-year-old is admitted into the hospital with a suspected diagnosis of acute renal failure. Which clinical findings should the nurse expect to observe? *(Choose all that apply.)*
   a. Metabolic acidosis and increased serum potassium
   b. Oliguria and elevated blood urea nitrogen levels
   c. Edema and proteinuria
   d. Bloody diarrhea and a positive test for *Escherichia coli*
   e. Fatigue and hypertension
   f. Decreased appetite and lethargy

7. A pale, listless 5-year-old is brought to the emergency department. The child has many bruises, decreased urine output, and bloody diarrhea. The nurse plans emergency care based on suspicion of:
   a. child abuse.
   b. glomerulonephritis.
   c. hemolytic uremic syndrome.
   d. hemorrhagic shock.

8. The most common cause of chronic renal failure in young children is:
   a. congenital renal abnormalities.
   b. insulin-dependent diabetes.
   c. hemolytic uremic syndrome.
   d. nephrotoxic antibiotic use.

9. Corticosteroids are used in the treatment of:
   a. glomerulonephritis.
   b. nephrotic syndrome.
   c. phimosis.
   d. vesicoureteral reflux.

10. In a child with end-stage renal disease, recombinant erythropoietin is used to treat:
    a. anemia.
    b. hypertension.
    c. rejection of a transplanted kidney.
    d. renal osteodystrophy.

11. The nurse is caring for a 10-year-old who was diagnosed with nephrotic syndrome. Which interventions should the nurse include in the child's plan of care? *(Choose all that apply.)*
    a. Obtain accurate weight every other day.
    b. Notify the physician if the urinary output is less than 4 mL/kg/hr.
    c. Ensure position changes every 2 hours.
    d. Monitor for fever, cough or abdominal pain.
    e. Adhere to no-added-salt diet.

12. The nurse is teaching a parent about home care for an 8-month-old who recently had surgical repair of hypospadias. Which statement made by the parent would indicate a correct understanding of the teaching?
    a. "I should monitor my infant's urine for cloudiness or a foul smell."
    b. "I should expect my infant to have a minimal amount of pain."
    c. "I should give my infant a smaller amount of formula in the bottle to limit the intake."
    d. "I should allow my infant to play on the floor as long as my infant does not cry."

13. The nurse is teaching a group of new pediatric nurses about disorders and anomalies of the genitourinary tract in children. Which statement made by one of the new nurses would indicate a need for additional teaching?
    a. "Hydrocele is a painless swelling of the scrotum caused by a collection of fluid."
    b. "Testicular torsion is a progressive condition that develops over a few days."
    c. "Phimosis can be corrected through cleaning and gentle manual retraction of the prepuce."
    d. "Bladder exstrophy needs to be covered with a non-adhesive plastic wrap until surgery is done."

21 The Child with a Respiratory Alteration

HELPFUL HINT

Review the anatomy and physiology of the respiratory system in an anatomy and physiology textbook.

STUDENT LEARNING EXERCISES

Definitions

Match each term with its definition.

1. _____ Atelectasis

2. _____ Crackles

3. _____ Dysphagia

4. _____ Dyspnea

5. _____ Grunting

6. _____ Hypercapnia

7. _____ Hypocapnia

8. _____ Hypoxemia

9. _____ Hypoxia

10. _____ Nasal flaring

11. _____ Nasal polyps

12. _____ Orthopnea

13. _____ Retractions

14. _____ Rhonchi

15. _____ Stridor

16. _____ Tachypnea

17. _____ Wheezing

a. Abnormal movements of the chest wall during inspiration
b. Sound, similar to a grunting noise, that can be heard with or without a stethoscope
c. Shrill, harsh sound heard during inspiration, expiration, or both
d. Increased respiratory rate
e. Widening of the nares that indicates air hunger
f. Increased levels of carbon dioxide in the blood
g. Difficulty breathing except in an upright position
h. Collapsed or airless part of the lung
i. High-pitched musical whistles heard with or without a stethoscope
j. Breath sounds caused by passage of air through thick secretions
k. Difficulty breathing
l. Decreased levels of carbon dioxide in the blood
m. Rales
n. Decreased oxygenation of cells and tissues
o. Decreased levels of oxygen in the blood
p. Difficulty swallowing
q. Semitransparent herniations of respiratory epithelium

Review of the Respiratory System and Diagnostic Tests

Answer as either true (T) or false (F).

18. _____ Lack of surfactant places a preterm infant at risk for respiratory distress syndrome.

19. _____ Diffusion of gases takes place in the upper airway.

20. _____ The tonsils help filter circulating lymph fluid.

21. _____ Arterial blood gases are used mainly to assess acid-base balance.

22. _____ A sweat test is used to diagnose allergies.

23. _____ Pulse oximetry is used to measure oxygen saturation.

Allergic Rhinitis

24. The onset of allergic rhinitis rarely occurs before age _____.

25. Classic manifestations of allergic rhinitis include: _____

_____

_____

26. Describe how parents can prepare saline solutions. _____

_____

Sinusitis

27. Acute sinusitis often follows a(n) _____.

28. Chronic sinusitis is associated with allergic rhinitis and _____.

29. Pain associated with sinusitis may be relieved by administering _____

and applying _____.

Otitis Media

Answer as either true (T) or false (F).

30. _____ Risk factors for otitis media include attending a day care center and bottle feeding.

31. _____ Ear drainage indicates otitis media with effusion.

32. _____ Tympanostomy tubes usually fall out spontaneously.

Pharyngitis and Tonsillitis

Answer as either true (T) or false (F).

33. _____ Children with allergies to penicillin are usually given erythromycin for viral pharyngitis.

34. _____ Abdominal pain and vomiting are manifestations of bacterial pharyngitis.

35. _____ Tonsillectomy reduces the incidence of recurrent pharyngitis.

Laryngomalacia

36. The hallmark of laryngomalacia is _____.

Croup

Match each type of croup with its description.

37. _____ Acute spasmodic croup

38. _____ Laryngotracheobronchitis

39. _____ Epiglottitis

40. _____ Tracheitis

a. Occurs more often in anxious, excitable children
b. Bacterial form of croup
c. Most common form of croup
d. Usually follows an upper respiratory infection

Answer as either true (T) or false (F).

41. _____ Children with laryngotracheobronchitis are typically afebrile.

42. _____ The Hib vaccine has reduced the incidence of tracheitis.

43. _____ Children who receive racemic epinephrine in the emergency department should be observed for at least 3 hours after treatment.

44. _____ Sedatives are frequently used to keep a child with croup calm.

Epiglottitis

45. Manifestations of epiglottitis include: _____.

_____

_____

46. When epiglottitis is suspected, never use a _____ to inspect the child's throat.

Bronchitis

47. Bronchitis is usually caused by a _____.

48. Treatment includes _____, _____, and _____.

Bronchiolitis

49. Respiratory syncytial virus (RSV) is the causative agent in bronchiolitis in more than _____ % of the cases.

50. Why is RSV so easily communicable? _____

_____

51. List the product that may be used monthly as RSV prophylaxis in preterm infants.

_____

Pneumonia

52. What can be done to promote pulmonary drainage in a child with pneumonia? _____

_____

_____

_____

53. The oxygen saturation of a child with pneumonia, who has no underlying chronic pulmonary disease, should be maintained at more than _____%.

Foreign Body Aspiration

54. List six foods that are commonly aspirated by young children.

a. _____

b. _____

c. _____

d. _____

e. _____

f. _____

55. Manifestations of an obstructed airway in a child who has aspirated are _____

and _____.

Pulmonary Noninfectious Irritation

56. Adult respiratory distress syndrome can be precipitated by _____

_____.

57. _____ is associated with increased respiratory infections in children.

58. _____ poisoning is a complication of smoke inhalation.

Respiratory Distress Syndrome

Answer as either true (T) or false (F).

59. _____ Respiratory distress syndrome (RDS) can result from inadequate amounts of surfactant.

60. _____ The incidence of RDS increases as gestational age increases.

61. _____ Central cyanosis is an early sign of RDS.

62. _____ Fluid replacement is used to both treat and prevent RDS.

Apnea

Match each term with its description.

63. _____ Apnea

64. _____ Periodic breathing

65. _____ Acute life-threatening event

    a. Three or more respiratory pauses lasting longer than 3 seconds with less than 20 seconds of respiration between pauses

    b. Cessation of breathing for at least 20 seconds, or for a shorter period if accompanied by bradycardia and cyanosis

    c. Sudden episode of apnea with changes in color and muscle tone accompanied by coughing or gagging

66. A nurse witnessing an apneic episode should note _____

_____

_____

_____.

67. When home apnea monitoring is prescribed, parents need instruction about _____

and _____.

Sudden Infant Death Syndrome

Answer as either true (T) or false (F).

68. _____ Sudden infant death syndrome (SIDS) usually occurs during sleep.

69. _____ SIDS usually occurs after the age of 6 months.

70. _____ Healthy infants should be placed supine for sleep.

71. _____ Most parents of an infant who has died from SIDS will feel guilt, anger, and emotional distress.

Asthma

72. In recent years the incidence and mortality rates for asthma have both _____.

73. Wheezing is typically heard on _____.

74. Tachypnea _____ carbon dioxide levels in the blood.

75. Beta$_2$-adrenergic agonists are used to _____.

76. Increasingly severe asthma that does not respond to vigorous treatment is called

_____.

77. _____ is an ideal sport for children with asthma.

78. Corticosteroids are used during an acute asthma attack to _____.

79. Children with asthma monitor their condition at home by using _____.

80. Mast cell inhibitors are given 30 minutes before _____.

Bronchopulmonary Dysplasia/Chronic Lung Disease of Infancy

Answer as either true (T) or false (F).

81. _____ Bronchopulmonary dysplasia (BPD) results from lung injury related to receiving supplemental oxygen and mechanical ventilation.

82. _____ Pursing of the lips and nasal flaring are early signs of impending respiratory distress.

83. _____ Diuretics are used to treat hypertension related to BPD.

84. _____ Infants with BPD tend to have irreversible developmental delays.

Cystic Fibrosis

Answer as either true (T) or false (F).

85. _____ Cystic fibrosis (CF) is an autosomal dominant inherited disorder.

86. _____ CF affects the functioning of the exocrine glands.

87. _____ Children with CF have malnutrition because of poor diet.

88. _____ Meconium ileus may be the first indicator of CF.

89. _____ Aerosolized antibiotics may be used in place of intravenous antibiotics.

90. _____ Aerobic exercise may be as effective as chest physiotherapy in relieving pulmonary obstruction in CF.

91. _____ Enzyme dosage is adjusted according to weight gain.

92. _____ A child with CF requires extra salt and fluids when the weather is hot.

Tuberculosis

Match each term with its description.

93. _____ Tuberculosis (TB) exposure

94. _____ TB infection

95. _____ TB disease

a. Recent contact with a person who has contagious TB
b. Positive skin test with signs and symptoms of TB
c. Positive skin test with no signs and symptoms of TB

Answer as either true (T) or false (F).

96. _____ Children with TB are rarely contagious.

97. _____ The Mantoux test is the preferred method of screening for TB.

98. _____ Children with TB infection are treated with the *Bacillus Calmette-Guérin* for 9 months.

99. _____ In infants, a negative tuberculin skin test rules out TB infection.

SUGGESTED LEARNING ACTIVITIES

1. Interview a public health nurse about the incidence of TB in your community. Has your community seen an increase in new cases of TB? If yes, to what does the nurse attribute this increase? Share your findings with the class.

2. Investigate an asthma self-help group for children in your community. How does it meet the child's informational and psychosocial needs? Report your findings to your class.

STUDENT LEARNING APPLICATIONS

Enhance your learning by discussing your answers with other students.

Parents bring their 2-month-old daughter, Tina, to the pediatrician. They are very anxious because she cries all the time and hasn't been eating or sleeping. They also tell you that she feels very hot. Tina is diagnosed with acute otitis media and given a prescription for 10 days of amoxicillin.

1. What would you teach the parents about the causes, risk factors, and course of acute otitis media?

2. What would you teach them about the treatment and follow-up?

Tina's parents remain extremely anxious. Their anxiety seems out of proportion to the situation. You are tempted to say, "It's just an ear infection. Lighten up."

3. Why would you *not say* that?

4. Why do you think the parents are so upset?

5. How can you determine whether you are correct?

In talking with Tina's parents, you discover that both of them had siblings who died before their first birthdays.

6. How does this information change your perception of their anxiety?

7. How can you effectively intervene with this family?

REVIEW QUESTIONS

Choose the best answer.

1. A toddler is admitted to the hospital with croup. The child is tachypneic with substernal retracting and nasal flaring, has a harsh, barking cough, and a pulse oximetry reading on room air of 98%. The most accurate nursing diagnosis for this child is:
   a. ineffective breathing pattern.
   b. ineffective airway clearance.
   c. impaired gas exchange.
   d. all of the above.

2. When preparing a 6-year-old child for a tonsillectomy the nurse should not:
   a. direct the teaching at the child's parents.
   b. reassure the child that he or she will be able to talk after the surgery.
   c. explain that his or her throat will be sore after surgery.
   d. explain that he or she will have to drink a lot after surgery.

3. An anxious and irritable preschooler arrives in the emergency department, refusing to lie down to be examined. The child sits up, leans forward onto the hands, and drools saliva. The child is warm to the touch and pale in color. The nurse should:
   a. take the child's vital signs.
   b. notify the physician immediately.
   c. ask the parents to wait outside the examining room.
   d. start an intravenous line.

Chapter **21** **The Child with a Respiratory Alteration**

4. Parents bring their 8-month-old son to the emergency department because, according to them, he's breathing so fast that he can't eat, and he feels hot. Physical examination reveals nasal flaring, intercostal retracting, and moderate expiratory wheezing. The nurse suspects that the infant has:
   a. acute spasmodic croup.
   b. bronchiolitis.
   c. epiglottitis.
   d. aspirated a foreign body.

5. The nurse is preparing a child for a bronchoscopy. The child most likely has:
   a. apnea.
   b. bronchiolitis.
   c. aspirated a foreign body.
   d. pneumonia.

6. Which drug is a respiratory stimulant?
   a. Isoniazid
   b. Albuterol
   c. Caffeine
   d. Ribavirin

7. Active bleeding in a child after a tonsillectomy is indicated by:
   a. refusal to drink fluids.
   b. frequent swallowing.
   c. "coffee grounds" emesis.
   d. all of the above.

8. A child has bronchoconstriction 5 hours after an acute asthma attack. This is an example of which kind of inflammatory response?
   a. Immediate
   b. Intermediate
   c. Delayed

9. The nurse is teaching a family about the use of pancreatic enzymes in the treatment of cystic fibrosis. What information should the nurse include? *(Choose all that apply.)*
   a. Give the preparation with every meal and snack.
   b. Dissolve the enzymes in warm whole milk.
   c. Increase the dosage if the child has loose, fatty stools.
   d. Chewing the enzymes will increase their efficacy.
   e. Skip a dose if the child is ill with a sore throat.

10. A test used in the diagnosis of cystic fibrosis is:
    a. RAST.
    b. sweat chloride.
    c. culture for *Pseudomonas*.
    d. Mantoux.

11. Which therapy is least likely to be used for a child with cystic fibrosis who is in the hospital with a respiratory infection?
    a. Chest physiotherapy every 3 hours
    b. Intravenous antibiotics
    c. Cough suppressant medications
    d. Postural drainage

12. An infant is hospitalized after an acute life-threatening event. The apnea monitor alarm suddenly sounds. The nurse should first:
    a. assess the infant.
    b. question witnesses about the triggering event.
    c. initiate CPR.
    d. reset the monitor.

13. The nurse is teaching a 14-year-old how to monitor asthma using a peak flow meter. Place in the correct order the steps for using a peak flow meter.
    a. Take a few deep breaths then slowly take the deepest breath possible.
    b. Repeat two more times, waiting 10 seconds between attempts.
    c. Blow out as hard and fast as possible with a short, sharp blast.
    d. Move the pointer on the meter to 0 and hold it horizontally.
    e. Place the mouthpiece on your tongue and close lips tightly around it.
    f. Record the highest of the three attempts.

14. The nurse is preparing an in-service on the classification of asthma severity. What information should the nurse include in the teaching? *(Choose all that apply.)*
    a. A child with intermittent asthma has symptoms that occur three times a week.
    b. A child with intermittent asthma does not miss school or have limitations with activities.
    c. A child with mild, persistent asthma has exacerbations that require a burst of oral corticosteroids.
    d. A child with moderate, persistent asthma has sleep disturbances more than once a week.
    e. A child with severe, persistent asthma has a PEFR that is less than 70% of predicted baseline.
    f. A child with severe, persistent asthma should use a bronchodilator several times a day.

15. The nurse is caring for an 18-month-old with a suspected case of acute tracheitis. What clinical manifestations would the nurse expect to observe? *(Choose all that apply.)*
    a. High fever
    b. Cough with purulent secretions
    c. Decreased breath sounds
    d. Inspiratory stridor
    e. Upper respiratory infection
    f. Audible wheezing

16. The nurse is teaching a parent of a 2-month-old who was born prematurely about safe use of oxygen at home. Which statement made by the parent indicates a correct understanding of the teaching?
    a. "I should keep a fire extinguisher on each floor of our house."
    b. "I should use petroleum jelly on my baby's lips to prevent dryness."
    c. "I should keep the oxygen tank lying flat on the floor in the baby's room."
    d. "I should keep the oxygen tank 5 to 6 feet from the space heater in the living room."

22 The Child with a Cardiovascular Alteration

Review the anatomy and physiology of the heart and fetal circulation in an anatomy and physiology textbook.

STUDENT LEARNING EXERCISES

Definitions

Match each term with its definition.

1. _____ Angioplasty

2. _____ Cardiomegaly

3. _____ Compensation

4. _____ Decompensation

5. _____ Arrhythmia

6. _____ Palpitation

7. _____ Pulmonary edema

8. _____ Pulmonary hypertension

9. _____ Pulmonary venous congestion

10. _____ Shunt

11. _____ Systemic venous congestion

12. _____ Valvuloplasty

a. Increased systemic venous pressure leading to excessive fluid in the systemic veins
b. Abnormal blood flow from one part of the circulatory system to another
c. Abnormal rhythm of the heart
d. Maintenance of adequate blood flow accomplished by cardiac and circulatory adjustments
e. Procedure to open a valve
f. Increased pulmonary pressure leading to excessive fluid in the pulmonary veins
g. Enlarged heart
h. Collection of excess fluid in alveoli
i. Sensation of rapid or irregular heartbeat
j. Inability of the heart to maintain adequate circulation
k. Increased pressure in pulmonary arteries and arterioles
l. Procedure that dilates vessels

Recall the definitions of the terms in italics in the following statements. Then, apply your knowledge and determine whether each statement is true (T) or false (F).

13. _____ *Central venous* pressure (CVP) is measured in the right ventricle.

14. _____ A drug's *chronotropic* effect has an impact on the heart's rate.

15. _____ A drug's *inotropic* effect has an impact on the heart's contractility.

16. _____ *Myocardial contractility* refers to the heart muscle's ability to shorten.

17. _____ *Afterload* is measured by determining CVP.

18. _____ *Pulmonary vascular resistance* affects the left ventricle.

19. _____ *Regurgitation* is turbulent blood flow.

20. _____ *Systemic vascular resistance* is the amount of pressure exerted by the systemic vascular bed.

21. _____ A *valvotomy* is a surgically created opening in a valve.

22. _____ Diseased tissue can be removed by *ablation*.

Review of the Cardiovascular System

Fill in the blanks.

23. In fetal circulation, gas exchange occurs in the _____.

24. In fetal circulation, oxygenated blood from the placenta flows from the right atrium into the left atrium through the

_____.

25. After birth, the fetal shunt between the pulmonary artery and the aorta, which is called the

_____, closes.

26. After birth, pulmonary vascular resistance _____ because the systemic arterial pressure

_____.

Cardiovascular Assessment

Answer as either true (T) or false (F).

27. _____ Clubbing of nail beds indicates chronic hypoxia.

28. _____ A gallop is a missing heart sound.

29. _____ The point of maximal impulse at the seventh intercostal space indicates cardiomegaly.

30. _____ Cool extremities in a warm room may indicate decreased cardiac output.

31. _____ Dyspnea is an indicator of congestive heart failure.

32. _____ Functional murmurs are indicators of heart abnormalities.

33. _____ Squatting is an attempt to improve hypoxia.

34. _____ Acrocyanosis in the neonate is an abnormal finding.

35. _____ Friction rubs are associated with inflammation.

36. _____ Poor weight gain is frequently associated with cardiac disease in children.

37. _____ Clicks are indicators of blockages in the coronary arteries.

38. _____ The heart sound S1 is heard best at the base of the heart.

39. _____ A thrill is a murmur that can be palpated.

40. _____ Normal capillary refill time is less than 2 seconds.

41. _____ Cardiac catheterization can be an interventional as well as a diagnostic procedure.

Physiologic Consequences of Congenital Heart Disease

42. In infants, early manifestations of congestive heart failure include: _____

_____.

Match each drug or class of drugs with its description.

43. _____ Furosemide

44. _____ Spironolactone

45. _____ Thiazide diuretic

46. _____ Digoxin

47. _____ Vasodilator

a. Acts on distal renal tubules
b. Potassium-sparing diuretic
c. Relaxes smooth muscles; decreases after-load
d. Increases cardiac output; has positive inotropic and negative chronotropic effects
e. Potent loop diuretic

48. In an infant, fluid retention is monitored by _____.

49. Before administering digoxin, the nurse should count _____, check

_____, and observe _____.

Answer as either true (T) or false (F).

50. _____ In Eisenmenger syndrome, an acyanotic defect with left-to-right shunting becomes a cyanotic defect with right-to-left shunting.

51. _____ Primary pulmonary hypertension can be associated with collagen disease.

52. _____ Children with left-to-right shunting have irreversible pulmonary hypertension.

Fill in the blanks.

53. Cyanosis typically occurs when oxygen saturation falls below _____%.

54. Explain how polycythemia compensates for chronic hypoxia. _____

_____

_____

55. Treatment of hypercyanotic episodes, or tet spells, include: _____

_____.

Left-to-Right Shunting Lesions

56. Patent ductus arteriosus is managed medically with _____.

57. Classic signs of _____ are decreased pulses and blood pressure in the lower extremities.

58. _____ is an abnormal opening between the ventricles, whereas

_____ is an abnormal opening between the atria.

59. Endocardial cushion defect is also known as _____.

60. Narrowing of the pulmonary artery is called _____.

61. Thickening of the aortic valve is known as _____.

Cyanotic Lesions with Increased or Decreased Pulmonary Blood Flow

Match each defect with its description.

62. _____ Transposition of the great arteries

63. _____ Hypoplastic left heart syndrome

64. _____ Pulmonary atresia

65. _____ Tetralogy of Fallot

66. _____ Tricuspid atresia

67. _____ Truncus arteriosus

68. _____ Total anomalous pulmonary venous return

a. Defect composed of four distinct lesions
b. Condition in which pulmonary artery and aorta are one vessel
c. Failure of the pulmonary valve to develop
d. Absence of tricuspid valve
e. Inadequate development of left side of the heart
f. Reversal of the aorta and the pulmonary artery
g. Absence of communication between the pulmonary veins and the left atrium

Infective Endocarditis, Rheumatic Fever, and Kawasaki Disease

Answer as either true (T) or false (F).

69. _____ Children with congenital heart disease have an increased risk for development of infective endocarditis.

70. _____ Endocarditis prophylaxis generally consists of an antibiotic taken orally 1 hour before invasive procedures.

71. _____ Immune complexes seem to play a role in infective endocarditis.

72. _____ Kawasaki disease is an immune-mediated condition resulting in vasculitis.

73. _____ Antibiotic prophylaxis with penicillin for at least 5 years is part of the management of rheumatic fever without cardiac complications.

74. _____ Vegetation seen on an echocardiogram suggests Kawasaki disease.

75. _____ Tetralogy of Fallot requires endocarditis prophylaxis.

76. _____ Kawasaki disease is associated with untreated or partially treated streptococcal infections.

77. _____ Manifestations of rheumatic fever include arthritis, carditis, chorea, heart murmur, and painless, red skin lesions.

Hypertension

Answer as either true (T) or false (F).

78. _____ Normal blood pressure for a child is defined as a systolic or diastolic blood pressure less than the 90th percentile for age and sex.

79. _____ Children with essential hypertension often have a family history of the disease.

80. _____ Renal disease is a complication of secondary hypertension.

81. _____ Steroids and oral contraceptives can cause hypertension.

82. _____ Secondary hypertension occurs more often in adolescents than in younger children.

83. _____ Nonpharmacologic therapies for primary hypertension are usually not effective in children and adolescents.

Cardiomyopathies

84. Which type of cardiomyopathy is a major cause of sudden cardiac death in adolescents?

_____

85. Which type results from an infection or exposure to a toxin? _____

_____

86. Drugs used to decrease ventricular hypercontractility and outflow tract obstruction are _____

and _____ blockers.

Arrhythmias

87. _____ is the most common primary symptomatic arrhythmia seen in children.

88. _____ is a major cause of bradycardia in children.

89. In _____, there is no cardiac output.

90. In asystole, _____ is administered to stimulate cardiac activity.

High Cholesterol Levels in Children and Adolescents

91. Risk factors for high cholesterol levels in children and adolescents include: _____

_____

_____.

92. In children, borderline levels for low-density lipoprotein cholesterol are _____ mg/dL, and a high

level is greater than _____ mg/dL.

SUGGESTED LEARNING ACTIVITIES

1. Role play with two other students. One student will act as the nurse and another student will be a parent, who has just learned that his or her child has a cardiac defect and will require surgery. The third student will observe the interaction. After 10 minutes, discuss the scenario. The nurse can describe how it felt to deal with the parent. The parent can describe which of the nurse's interventions were effective and which could be improved. The observer can describe the interchange from an objective viewpoint.

2. Interview the parent of a child who has had cardiac surgery in the past. Try to discover what the health care team did that was helpful for the family during the child's hospitalization. What could have been done better?

3. Observe a cardiac catheterization. Design a plan that teaches a 12-year-old child what to expect during catheterization.

STUDENT LEARNING APPLICATIONS

Enhance your learning by discussing your answers with other students.

Michael is a healthy 10 year old undergoing a routine physical examination. His height and weight are at the 75th percentile. His blood pressure is at the 95th percentile for his age and sex, but a review of his chart reveals that his blood pressure has been slightly below the 90th percentile on previous visits.

1. On the basis of these findings, what questions would you ask Michael and his parents?

_____

_____

2. How would you further assess his blood pressure?

_____

The physician makes the diagnosis of essential hypertension and decides to initiate nonpharmacologic therapy.

3. How would you assess the family's need for information about the following treatments?

    a. Weight control _____

    b. Physical conditioning _____

    c. Dietary modifications _____

    d. Relaxation techniques _____

4. What key features of these treatments would you stress when you present the information?

5. How would you evaluate the effectiveness of your presentation?

REVIEW QUESTIONS

Choose the best answer.

1. In the physical assessment of an infant with a ventricular septal defect (VSD), the nurse notices hepatosplenomegaly and periorbital edema. He understands that these are clinical manifestations of:
   a. heart failure.
   b. endocarditis.
   c. fluid overload.
   d. decreased central venous pressure.

2. Percentiles for average blood pressure are based on a child's:
   a. weight and sex.
   b. age and sex.
   c. sex and race.
   d. age and weight.

3. The nurse is caring for an infant with cardiovascular alterations. Which nursing interventions would be appropriate to include in the child's plan of care? *(Choose all that apply.)*
   a. Discouraging breastfeeding
   b. Limiting bottle feedings to 20 to 30 minutes
   c. Maintaining a neutral thermal environment
   d. Providing periods of uninterrupted rest
   e. Administering low-dose aspirin two times per day

4. Children with hypertension who are receiving loop diuretics are at risk for imbalances of:
   a. calcium.
   b. chloride.
   c. potassium.
   d. sodium.

5. A toddler is hospitalized with congestive heart failure and is receiving digoxin and furosemide. The child vomited twice in the past 4 hours. The nurse's best action is to:
   a. increase the child's fluid intake.
   b. omit the next dose of furosemide.
   c. check the child's blood pressure before the next dose of digoxin.
   d. get an order to draw a digoxin level.

6. An infant with a left-to-right shunt is admitted to the hospital in congestive heart failure. Yesterday, the child weighed 3.6 kg. Which clinical findings would indicate a worsening of the child's condition? *(Choose all that apply.)*
   a. Weight of 3.7 kg
   b. Urine output of 40 mL in the past 8 hours
   c. Rales in the lower lobes
   d. Blood pressure of 102/64 mm Hg
   e. Respiratory rate of 58 breaths per minute
   f. Increased irritability

7. While doing a newborn assessment, the nurse finds the infant's blood pressure in the arms is much higher than in the legs. The nurse suspects that the infant has:
   a. aortic stenosis.
   b. endocardial cushion defect.
   c. coarctation of the aorta.
   d. truncus arteriosus.

8. Parents of a toddler with tetralogy of Fallot explain that because they do not want the child to become overexerted, they confine the child in a playpen or crib to limit mobility. On the basis of this information, the most appropriate nursing diagnosis is:
   a. Activity Intolerance.
   b. Risk for Altered Parenting.
   c. Caregiver Role Strain.
   d. Risk for Altered Growth and Development.

9. While taking routine vital signs, the nurse notices the infant is having a hypercyanotic episode. What should the nurse do first?
   a. Continue getting vital signs for a baseline comparison.
   b. Place the infant in a knee-chest position.
   c. Get a pulse oximetry reading.
   d. Give the child morphine sulfate.

10. Parents of children with congenital heart problems often feel a loss of control when the child is hospitalized. The nurse who understands this will:
    a. encourage parents to participate in their child's care.
    b. explain procedures before performing them.
    c. answer questions honestly.
    d. all of the above.

11. The father of a child with a congenital heart defect asks the nurse why his daughter has to take penicillin before she gets her teeth cleaned by the dentist. The nurse explains that this is necessary to prevent:
    a. infective endocarditis.
    b. congestive heart failure.
    c. rheumatic fever.
    d. infected gums.

12. What is an indicator of infective endocarditis?
    a. Positive blood cultures
    b. Vegetation seen on Holter monitoring
    c. Decreased erythrocyte sedimentation rate
    d. All of the above

13. The nurse is preparing an in-service about rheumatic fever for a group of pediatric nurses. What information should the nurse include in the teaching? *(Choose all that apply.)*
    a. Rheumatic fever is diagnosed by using the Jones criteria in the presence of at least two major characteristics or one major and two minor manifestations.
    b. Rheumatic fever manifests in 2 to 6 weeks after an untreated or partially treated group A beta-hemolytic streptococcal infection of the upper respiratory tract.
    c. Rheumatic fever is a prevalent condition that is epidemic in the southwest regions of the United States.
    d. Rheumatic fever occurs once in a lifetime but can have significant long-term cardiac involvement.
    e. Rheumatic fever has clinical manifestations including arthritis, carditis, and chorea.
    f. Rheumatic fever is treated with a 10-day course of oral penicillin, anti-inflammatory agents, and bed rest.

14. The nurse is teaching a parent of a 3-year-old who had heart surgery 5 days ago about care after discharge. Which statement made by the parent would indicate a correct understanding of the teaching?
    a. "I should call the physician daily with my child's weight and temperature."
    b. "I should apply lotion to my child's scar to reduce scarring."
    c. "I should limit my child's fluid intake until the first check-up."
    d. "I should allow my child to resume regular quiet activities."

15. The nurse is preparing to admit a 2-year-old with tetralogy of Fallot. Which clinical manifestations would the nurse expect to find? *(Choose all that apply.)*
    a. Boot-shaped heart on radiography
    b. Harsh systolic murmur with a palpable thrill
    c. Chronic hypoxemia
    d. Poor lower extremity peripheral perfusion
    e. Profound central cyanosis

23 The Child with a Hematologic Alteration

HELPFUL HINT

Review the anatomy and physiology of the hematologic system in an anatomy and physiology textbook.

STUDENT LEARNING EXERCISES

Definitions

Match each term with its definition.

1. _____ Autoimmune disorder

2. _____ Chelation

3. _____ Erythropoiesis

4. _____ Extramedullary

5. _____ Granulocytes

6. _____ Hematopoiesis

7. _____ Hemolysis

8. _____ Hemosiderosis

9. _____ Pancytopenia

10. _____ Reticulocytes

11. _____ Reticuloendothelial system

a. Outside the bone marrow
b. Collection of cells capable of phagocytosis
c. Reduction in all types of blood cells
d. Breakdown of red blood cells
e. Increase in tissue iron stores
f. Production of red blood cells
g. Immature red blood cells
h. Production of blood cells
i. Disorder in which the body launches an immunologic response against itself
j. Neutrophils, eosinophils, or basophils
k. Binding of a metallic ion with a structure that results in inactivation of the ion

Review of the Hematologic System

12. Explain the function of:

   a. Red blood cells: _____

   b. White blood cells: _____

   c. Platelets: _____

13. Define each term:

   a. Anemia: _____

   b. Polycythemia: _____

    c. Lymphopenia:_____

    d. Megakaryocytes:_____

Iron Deficiency Anemia

14. How does the introduction of cow's milk into the diet before 1 year of age affect the development of iron-deficiency anemia (IDA)?

_____

_____

15. Why are infants with IDA lethargic? _____

_____

16. Give two reasons why adolescents are prone to IDA.

    a. _____

    b. _____

17. What foods can interfere with iron absorption? _____

_____

_____

Sickle Cell Disease

18. Under what three conditions do red blood cells change to a sickle shape?

    a. _____

    b. _____

    c. _____

19. Sickle cells cause vaso-occlusion. What does this lead to? _____

_____

Match each complication of sickle cell disease with its clinical manifestation

20. _____ Vaso-occlusive crisis

21. _____ Acute chest syndrome

22. _____ Dactylitis

23. _____ Stroke

24. _____ Acute splenic sequestration

25. _____ Aplastic anemia

26. _____ Priapism

    a. Altered level of consciousness
    b. Painful, persistent erection
    c. Pallor, lethargy, and fainting
    d. Swelling of hands and feet
    e. Signs of hypovolemic shock
    f. Fever, cough, and chest pain
    g. Severe pain

Chapter **23** **The Child with a Hematologic Alteration**

Beta-Thalassemia

27. Beta-thalassemia is inherited in a(n) _____ pattern.

28. The major complication of the treatment of beta-thalassemia is _____.

29. In beta-thalassemia, chelation removes _____ from the body.

30. The drug used to manage hemosiderosis is _____.

Hemophilia

31. Describe the parents of a girl with hemophilia. _____

_____

32. In hemophilia A, the missing blood clotting component is _____; in hemophilia B,

the missing component is _____.

33. What are the manifestations of bleeding into the joints? _____

_____

34. Hemophilia is a genetic disorder carried on the _____ chromosome.

von Willebrand Disease

Answer as either true (T) or false (F).

35. _____ von Willebrand disease is the most commonly acquired bleeding disorder.

36. _____ Prolonged and excessive bleeding and menorrhagia are signs of von Willebrand disease.

37. _____ The von Willebrand protein is a carrier protein for factor IX.

38. _____ The treatment of choice for von Willebrand disease type I and type IIA is desmopressin acetate.

Immune Thrombocytopenic Purpura

Answer as either true (T) or false (F).

39. _____ Immune thrombocytopenic purpura (ITP) results in the destruction and decreased production of the platelets.

40. _____ ITP is an autoimmune disorder.

41. _____ Petechiae and bruising are clinical manifestations of ITP.

42. _____ Splenectomy is the treatment of choice for ITP.

43. _____ ITP can be either an acute or a chronic disorder.

Disseminated Intravascular Coagulation

Answer as either true (T) or false (F).

44. _____ Excessive bleeding and excessive clotting occur at the same time in disseminated intravascular coagulation (DIC).

45. _____ In DIC, bleeding occurs because of the depletion of platelets and clotting factors.

46. _____ Excessive bruising and oozing from venipuncture sites are late signs of DIC.

Aplastic Anemia

47. In aplastic anemia, the bone marrow stops producing _____,

_____, and _____.

48. Clinical manifestations of aplastic anemia include: _____

_____

49. Medications used to treat aplastic anemia include steroids, cyclosporin, antithymocyte/anti-lymphocyte globulin,

and _____.

ABO Incompatibility and Hemolytic Diseases of the Newborn

50. ABO incompatibility results when the mother has blood type O and the fetus has either blood type _____ or

_____.

51. Rh incompatibility results when the maternal type is Rh _____ and the fetal type is Rh _____.

52. Rh incompatibility can be prevented by administering RhoGAM to Rh-negative mothers after:

_____

Hyperbilirubinemia

Answer as either true (T) or false (F).

53. _____ Neonatal hyperbilirubinemia is referred to as physiologic jaundice.

54. _____ Kernicterus refers to damage to liver cells.

55. _____ Hyperbilirubinemia is more common in term infants.

56. _____ Phototherapy allows unconjugated bilirubin to be removed by the liver and spleen.

57. _____ After an exchange transfusion, phototherapy is no longer necessary.

SUGGESTED LEARNING ACTIVITIES

With one or several other students in a discussion group, review the genetic implications of inherited hematologic disorders by discussing the following questions.

1. Sickle cell disease is an autosomal recessive disorder.

   a. When both parents have the trait, what are the chances that:

      (1) A child will have neither the trait nor the disease? _____

      (2) A child will have the disease? _____

      (3) A child will have the trait? _____

Chapter **23** **The Child with a Hematologic Alteration**

b. When one parent has the disease and the other has the trait, what are the chances that:

(1) A child will have neither the trait nor the disease? _____

(2) A child will have the disease? _____

(3) A child will have the trait? _____

c. When neither parent has the disease but one has the trait, what are the chances that:

(1) A child will have neither the trait nor the disease? _____

(2) A child will have the disease? _____

(3) A child will have the trait? _____

2. Hemophilia is an inherited X-linked recessive disorder.

a. When the mother is a carrier and the father does not have hemophilia, what are the chances that:

(1) A daughter will have the disease? _____

(2) A daughter will be a carrier? _____

(3) A son will have the disease? _____

(4) A son will be a carrier? _____

b. When the mother is a carrier and the father has hemophilia, what are the chances that:

(1) A daughter will have the disease? _____

(2) A daughter will be a carrier? _____

(3) A son will have the disease? _____

(4) A son will be a carrier? _____

STUDENT LEARNING APPLICATIONS

Enhance your learning by discussing your answers with other students.

Joellen is a 12-year-old girl admitted to the hospital in a vaso-occlusive sickle cell crisis. Her pain is localized in her right arm and shoulder, and she rates it as 3.5 on a 0 to 5 scale. Her vital signs are slightly elevated, with her oral temperature at 100.7 F. She weighs 40 kg.

1. Joellen is receiving morphine sulfate for pain. As her nurse, what nonpharmacologic measures for pain management might you also use for Joellen?

The physician orders IV fluids for Joellen to run at 2× maintenance.

2. What are Joellen's basic fluid maintenance requirements for a 24-hour period? What should her hourly IV rate be to provide 2× maintenance fluids?

3. You want to assess Joellen's knowledge about prevention of sickle cell crises. How would you do this?

4. While caring for Joellen, you notice that she has a productive cough. She also starts to complain about pain in her chest. How would you address this new problem?

REVIEW QUESTIONS

Choose the best answer.

1. An example of an autoimmune disorder is:
   a. hemolytic disease of the newborn.
   b. disseminated vascular coagulation.
   c. immune thrombocytopenic purpura.
   d. von Willebrand disease.

2. If a preschooler with mild hemophilia has joint pain, the nurse should:
   a. administer children's aspirin.
   b. apply cold compresses.
   c. do passive range-of-motion exercises.
   d. give the child a warm bath in the tub.

3. Which of these statements about chelation therapy is true?
   a. It is used to rid the body of excess sulfate.
   b. It is used to treat one of the complications of factor VIII therapy.
   c. It is used to manage hemosiderosis.
   d. It often results in increased bleeding.

4. An example of a disorder inherited in an autosomal dominant pattern is:
   a. hemophilia A.
   b. beta-thalassemia.
   c. von Willebrand disease.
   d. ABO-Rh incompatibility.

5. Which statement made by an adolescent with iron-deficiency anemia indicates that he or she needs to review information about iron supplements?
   a. "I'll take my pill with orange juice."
   b. "I'll keep the pills out of reach of my younger brother and sister."
   c. "I'll double the dose during my periods."
   d. "I'll call the doctor if the pills upset my stomach."

6. Four-year-old Sara is admitted to the hospital with sickle cell disease. Her vital signs are as follows: Temperature is 99° F, heart rate is 124 beats per minute, respirations are 38/minute, and blood pressure is 70/40 mm Hg. She is pale and listless and has splenomegaly. She has:
   a. aplastic crisis.
   b. acute chest syndrome.
   c. a cerebrovascular accident.
   d. acute sequestration crisis.

7. An infant receiving phototherapy for hyperbilirubinemia is at increased risk for:
   a. hyperthermia.
   b. hypothermia.
   c. dehydration.
   d. all of the above.

8. A 6-year-old hospital patient complains of a headache. This could be a sign of a serious complication if the child has:
   a. aplastic anemia.
   b. hemophilia.
   c. sickle cell disease.
   d. any of the above.

9. A toddler with hemophilia is at risk for:
   a. altered growth related to poor appetite.
   b. developmental delay related to activity restrictions.
   c. infection related to decreased WBCs.
   d. all of the above.

10. When taking the history of a child with immune thrombocytopenic purpura (ITP), the nurse is not surprised to discover that:
    a. the child's father has classic hemophilia.
    b. the child had the flu 2 weeks ago.
    c. the child's grandmother has ITP.
    d. the child suddenly had a red, raised rash appear today.

11. The nurse is caring for four children on a pediatric unit. Which child should the nurse assess first?
    a. A 12-year-old with thalassemia who returned from a splenectomy 1 hour ago and is thirsty.
    b. A 10-year-old with sickle cell disease who is reporting chest pain.
    c. An 8-year-old with hemophilia who is reporting epistaxis.
    d. A 6-year-old with iron-deficiency anemia whose parent needs discharge instructions.

12. The nurse is caring for a child with disseminated intravascular coagulation. Which clinical findings would the nurse expect to observe? *(Choose all that apply.)*
    a. Decreased fibrinogen level
    b. High platelet count
    c. Purpuric rash
    d. Significant jaundice
    e. Oozing from puncture sites

24 The Child with Cancer

HELPFUL HINT

Review a pharmacology textbook for a more extensive discussion of chemotherapy.

STUDENT LEARNING EXERCISES

Definitions

Match each term with its definition.

1. _____ Benign

2. _____ Blast cell

3. _____ Clean margins

4. _____ Extramedullary

5. _____ Immunosuppression

6. _____ Intrathecal

7. _____ Malignant

8. _____ Neutropenia

9. _____ Protocol

10. _____ Thrombocytopenia

a. Immature lymphocytes
b. Plan of care outlining drug therapy and follow-up care
c. Within the spinal column
d. Decrease in number of cells, which results in reduced ability to fight infection
e. Reduction in platelet count
f. Slow-growing cells forming a tumor with distinct borders
g. Outside the bone marrow
h. Evidence of normal, disease-free tissue in the outermost layer of cells of a surgical sample
i. Abnormal cells that have invasive and unregulated growth
j. Weakening of the body's normal immune response

Review of Cancer

11. Any tumor that arises from new, abnormal growth is called a _____.

12. The two ways that cancer cells spread are _____ and _____.

13. Why is staging done for tumors? _____

_____

Answer as either true (T) or false (F).

14. _____ The cause of most childhood cancers is unknown.

15. _____ The cardinal signs of cancer in children are the same as in an adult.

16. _____ Screening tests are available for the detection of childhood cancers.

17. The signs and symptoms of childhood cancer depend on which factors? _____

_____.

18. Identify the three primary treatment modalities for children with cancer.

   a. _____

   b. _____

   c. _____

19. Chemotherapy is the use of _____ to kill cancer cells.

20. Identify the three body systems whose cells are most often affected by chemotherapy.

   a. _____

   b. _____

   c. _____

21. Define nadir. _____

_____

22. _____ places the child with cancer at risk for the development of opportunistic infections.

Identify each of the signs and symptoms as a side effect of chemotherapy (C), radiation (R), or both (B).

23. _____ Skin reactions

24. _____ Nausea and vomiting

25. _____ Alopecia

26. _____ Bone marrow suppression

27. _____ Stomatitis

28. _____ Fatigue

29. Which class of antiemetic drugs has been found to be most effective in treating chemotherapy-induced nausea and vomiting?

_____

30. What is the purpose of a biopsy in the treatment of childhood cancer? _____

_____

31. Why would a central venous catheter facilitate chemotherapy administration? _____

_____

32. The side effects of radiation therapy are specific to the _____ and

_____.

33. The side effects of radiation therapy usually appear _____ days after treatment is initiated.

34. _____ is the most common side effect of radiation therapy.

35. What is an autologous peripheral stem cell transplant? _____

_____

36. For what childhood cancers has bone marrow transplantation become standard therapy?

_____

37. What is conditioning? _____

38. The major problem associated with an allogenic transplant is _____.

39. What are biologic response modifiers? _____

_____

Leukemia

40. Leukemia is caused by the proliferation of _____.

41. List five clinical manifestations of leukemia.

a. _____

b. _____

c. _____

d. _____

e. _____

42. The diagnostic test that confirms a diagnosis of leukemia is _____.

43. The preferred treatment for leukemia is _____.

44. When is a child with acute lymphocytic leukemia considered to be in remission? _____

_____

45. Why are allopurinol and intravenous fluids with sodium bicarbonate given before chemotherapy? _____

_____

46. List five nursing diagnoses for the child with leukemia.

a. _____

b. _____

c. _____

d. _____

e. _____

47. Why are rectal temperatures contraindicated in the child with neutropenia? _____

_____

48. A child is at severe risk of infection when his or her absolute neutrophil level is _____.

49. What should the nurse teach the child with leukemia and family about oral hygiene?

_____

50. Why are live-virus vaccines contraindicated for the child with leukemia? _____

_____

51. What action is indicated if an immunosuppressed child is exposed to someone with varicella? _____

_____

52. What precautions should be taken for a child who is thrombocytopenic? _____

_____

53. What types of foods or fluids should be offered to the child who is nauseated? _____

_____

Answer as either true (T) or false (F).

54. _____ When a child is nauseated, warm liquids are better tolerated than cold liquids.

55. _____ Offering the child his favorite food will distract a child from his nausea.

56. _____ Hair may grow back a different color and texture after chemotherapy.

57. _____ Skin that is erythematous as a result of radiation can be massaged with any type of lotion.

58. _____ Oral temperatures are contraindicated for the child with mouth ulcers.

Brain Tumors

59. Manifestations of brain tumors vary with _____ and _____.

60. What are the two hallmark symptoms of brain tumors in children? _____

_____

61. The imaging modality most commonly used to evaluate brain tumors is _____.

62. Which treatment modalities are used to treat brain tumors in children? _____

_____

63. Why is Trendelenburg's position contraindicated after a craniotomy? _____

_____

64. Postoperatively after resection of a brain tumor, it is important for the nurse to assess a child for signs of:

_____.

Other Childhood Cancers

Answer as either true (T) or false (F).

65. _____ Lymphomas are the most common solid tumors occurring in children.

66. _____ The abdominal mass in a child with Wilms tumor should be palpated every shift for changes.

67. _____ Treatment for tumor lysis syndrome includes allopurinol and hydration with intravenous fluids containing sodium bicarbonate.

68. _____ The primary treatment modality for non-Hodgkin lymphoma is surgery.

69. _____ Neuroblastoma is a solid tumor that is found in infants and children.

70. _____ In the majority of cases, neuroblastoma manifests as a primary abdominal mass.

71. _____ Ewing sarcoma is the most common primary bone malignancy in children.

72. _____ Treatment of osteogenic sarcoma involves surgery and chemotherapy.

73. _____ A common manifestation of retinoblastoma is leukocoria.

CREATE YOUR OWN STUDY GUIDE

Provide the description/pathophysiologic information for each condition or tumor listed in the following table.

	Description/Pathophysiology
Wilms tumor	
Hodgkin disease	
Non-Hodgkin lymphoma	
Neuroblastoma	
Osteosarcoma	
Ewing sarcoma	
Rhabdomyosarcoma	
Retinoblastoma	

Describe the clinical manifestations and treatment for each condition or tumor listed in the following table.

	Clinical Manifestations	Therapeutic Interventions	Nursing Care Specific to the Condition or Treatment
Wilms tumor			
Hodgkin disease			
Non-Hodgkin lymphoma			
Neuroblastoma			
Osteosarcoma			
Ewing sarcoma			
Rhabdomyosarcoma			
Retinoblastoma			

SUGGESTED LEARNING ACTIVITIES

1. Investigate the guidelines for administration of chemotherapy at your clinical site.

2. If there is an oncology clinic at your clinical site, talk with the nurses about their responsibilities in the oncology clinic. Do the nurses need more advanced preparation in pediatric oncology?

STUDENT LEARNING APPLICATIONS

Enhance your learning by discussing your answers with other students.

The parents of 7-year-old Tom are concerned because he has had a low-grade fever for a week. His appetite and energy levels are decreased. They have also noticed bruises on Tom's legs although he has not been physically active. A complete blood cell count shows blast cells on the differential count. Tom is referred to a pediatric oncologist because leukemia is suspected; he is then admitted to the hospital. This is Tom's first day in the hospital, and you are caring for him.

1. What diagnostic studies would you expect to be ordered for Tom?

2. Respond to the following questions asked by Tom's father: "What is a bone marrow biopsy? Why does Tom need this test?"

When a bone marrow aspiration confirms acute lymphocytic leukemia, chemotherapy is initiated.

3. What are the nurse's responsibilities when caring for a child receiving chemotherapy?

4. What nursing assessments will you make while Tom is receiving chemotherapy?

When his parents leave the room to go to the cafeteria for lunch, Tom asks you several questions. How would you respond to his questions below?

5. "Do I have to have a transplant?"

6. "What are my chances?"

7. "How long do I have to get chemo?"

8. "Will I lose my hair?"

REVIEW QUESTIONS

Choose the best answer.

1. Bone marrow transplantation is considered standard therapy for which childhood cancer?
   a. Acute myelocytic leukemia
   b. Wilms tumor
   c. Osteosarcoma
   d. Hodgkin disease

2. The most common side effect of radiation therapy is:
   a. vomiting.
   b. bone marrow suppression.
   c. fatigue.
   d. erythema at the site.

3. Which position is contraindicated for a child after surgery to remove a brain tumor?
   a. Supine
   b. Prone
   c. Trendelenburg's
   d. Low Fowler's

4. When a child's own bone marrow is used in a bone marrow transplant, it is called a(n):
   a. allogenic transplant.
   b. autologous transplant.
   c. stem cell transplant.
   d. syngeneic transplant.

5. Which of the following is *not* a biologic response modifier?
   a. Monoclonal antibodies
   b. Interleukins
   c. Tumor necrosis factors
   d. Immunoglobulins

6. A child has a history of a fever of unknown origin, excessive bruising, and fatigue. This combination of symptoms is suggestive of which childhood cancer?
   a. Leukemia
   b. Neuroblastoma
   c. Lymphoma
   d. Osteosarcoma

7. A diagnosis of leukemia is confirmed by which study?
   a. Lumbar puncture
   b. Bone scan
   c. Bone marrow biopsy
   d. Complete blood cell count

8. Which precautions should be taken for a child with a platelet count of $18,000/mm^3$?
   a. Eat a low-bacteria diet.
   b. Use a soft-bristled toothbrush.
   c. Get extra rest.
   d. Start an iron supplement.

9. What is the best fluid for the child who is nauseated from chemotherapy?
   a. Milkshake in child's favorite flavor
   b. Room temperature water
   c. Sips of cold soda
   d. Hot tea with honey

10. What would the nurse tell an adolescent receiving chemotherapy about alopecia?
    a. "Don't worry. Most chemotherapy does not cause hair loss."
    b. "Your hair might grow back in a different color or texture."
    c. "Your hair will come back when you are finished with all your chemotherapy."
    d. "Aren't you lucky? The bald look is in right now."

11. Which intervention would be included in a plan of care for a child with Wilms tumor?
    a. Palpate the abdominal mass for any changes.
    b. Teach the child and family about a nephrectomy (key).
    c. Explain the need for radiation and surgery to remove the tumor to the family.
    d. Prepare the child for a bone-marrow aspiration.

12. The prevention of tumor lysis syndrome would include:
    a. hydration and alkalinizing the urine.
    b. administering sodium bicarbonate to make the urine acidic.
    c. assessing urine for hematuria.
    d. administering leukovorin rescue.

13. What is the risk for infection if a child's absolute neutrophil count is less than 400 cells/mm^3?
    a. Severe
    b. Moderate
    c. Minimal
    d. Not significant

14. What is considered a hallmark symptom of a brain tumor in children?
    a. Ataxia
    b. Morning vomiting
    c. Visual changes
    d. Seizure

15. The nurse recognizes which as an overt sign or symptom of childhood cancer?
    a. Whitish reflex in one eye
    b. An enlarged lymph node
    c. Change in bowel patterns
    d. Persistent headache

16. The nurse is caring for a 12-year-old who received radiation treatment 3 months ago and is being admitted for subacute side effects of radiation to the brain. Which side effects would the nurse expect to observe? *(Choose all that apply.)*
    a. Change in personality and behavior
    b. Fever and irritability
    c. Alopecia and vomiting
    d. Anorexia and dysphagia
    e. Mucositis and stomatitis
    f. Pronounced drowsiness and malaise

17. The nurse is teaching a parent with a child with cancer about home care after discharge. Which statement made by the parent would indicate a need for additional teaching?
    a. "I should administer acetaminophen to my child for pain or fever since my child is neutropenic."
    b. "I will complete a complete check on my child's oral mucous membranes for bleeding each day."
    c. "I should only allow the home health nurse to provide care to my child since I am not medically trained."
    d. "I will find time to attend the support group at the hospital or contact community resources after my child is discharged."

18. The nurse is preparing an in-service on pediatric brain tumors. What information should the nurse include? *(Choose all that apply.)*
    a. Clinical manifestations of a brain tumor in infants include lethargy and poor feeding.
    b. School-age children with a brain tumor will have intense headaches and insomnia.
    c. Many children with brain tumors have seizures, so seizure precautions should be initiated.
    d. After successful removal of a brain tumor the child will not exhibit signs of increased intracranial pressure.
    e. The child should not be told that his or her hair will be shaved until after the surgery is completed so as not to cause anxiety before the surgery.
    f. Parents of a child with a brain tumor need to be taught the side effects of both chemotherapy and radiation.

25 The Child with Major Alterations in Tissue Integrity

HELPFUL HINT

Review the topic of skin assessment in Chapter 9 and all of Chapter 15 in your textbook.

STUDENT LEARNING EXERCISES

Definitions

Match each term with its definition.

1. _____ Debridement
2. _____ Desquamation
3. _____ Ecchymosis
4. _____ Eschar
5. _____ Erythema
6. _____ Excoriation
7. _____ Intertrigo
8. _____ Keratosis
9. _____ Lichenification
10. _____ Pruritus
11. _____ Urticaria

a. Thickening and hardening of the skin
b. Scratch or abrasion of the skin
c. Itching
d. Sloughing of the skin in scales or sheets
e. Redness of the skin
f. Overgrowth and thickening of the cornified epithelium
g. Vascular reaction of the skin characterized by pruritic wheals
h. Dark plaque associated with tissue necrosis
i. Discoloration of skin or mucous membranes caused by leakage of blood into subcutaneous tissue
j. Maceration of two closely apposed skin surfaces
k. Removal of foreign material and devitalized or contaminated tissue from a traumatic or infected lesion to expose healthy tissue

Review of the Integumentary System

12. List the five major functions of the skin.

a. _____

b. _____

c. _____

d. _____

e. _____

Answer as either true (T) or false (F).

13. _____ The skin is a sensitive indicator of a child's general health.

14. _____ The epidermis is completely replaced every 4 weeks.

15. _____ A port-wine stain usually disappears after the first year of life.

16. _____ Vascular birthmarks are extremely uncommon.

Infections of the Skin

Impetigo

17. The most common skin infection of childhood is _____.

18. The organism responsible for most of the cases of impetigo is _____.

19. Describe the appearance of primary lesions of impetigo.

    a. Bullous: _____

    b. Crusted: _____

20. Failure to respond to treatment may indicate the infection is caused by which organism?

_____

21. What is the treatment for impetigo? _____

_____

22. What is a complication of impetigo caused by beta-hemolytic streptococci? _____

_____

23. What should parents be taught about preventing the spread of impetigo? _____

_____

Cellulitis

24. What is cellulitis? _____

_____

25. Which areas of the body are most commonly affected by cellulitis? _____

_____

26. Name three clinical manifestations of cellulitis.

    a. _____

    b _____

    c. _____

Chapter **25** **The Child with Major Alterations in Tissue Integrity**

27. How is cellulitis treated? _____

_____

28. Identify four nursing interventions for a child with cellulitis on his lower leg.

    a. _____

    b. _____

    c. _____

    d. _____

Candidiasis

29. What is the organism responsible for causing thrush? _____

_____

30. Describe the clinical manifestations of thrush. _____

_____

31. What questions should the nurse ask the mother of an infant with oral candidiasis during an assessment?

_____

_____

_____

32. The medication used to treat oral candidiasis is _____.

33. How should the prescribed medication be administered to an infant with oral candidiasis?

_____

_____

Tinea Infections

34. Identify the body parts affected in the following tinea infections.

    a. Tinea capitis: _____

    b. Tinea corporis: _____

    c. Tinea pedis: _____

35. What medications are used in the treatment of the following tinea infections, and how are they administered?

    a. Tinea capitis: _____

    b. Tinea corporis: _____

c. Tinea cruris: _____

d. Tinea pedis: _____

Answer as either true (T) or false (F).

36. _____ Tinea occurs when fungus invades the hair, the stratum corneum layer of the skin, or the nails.

37. _____ Tinea infections are not contagious to others.

38. _____ Tinea infections heal more quickly if the affected area is kept warm and moist.

Herpes Simplex Virus Infection

39. What is herpetic whitlow? _____

_____

40. What medication can lessen the severity of HSV-1? _____

41. How would a nurse advise a mother of a child with HSV-1 lesions on the lips who does not want to eat or drink?

_____

_____

Lice Infestations

Answer as either true (T) or false (F).

42. _____ Lice can be transmitted only by direct contact with an infested person.

43. _____ Clean hair is a deterrent to head lice.

Fill in the blanks.

44. Describe what the nurse is looking for when assessing a child for head lice. _____

_____

45. Give three interventions that should be taken if head lice are found.

a. _____

b. _____

c. _____

Mite Infestation (Scabies)

46. How is scabies transmitted? _____

_____

47. Name the clinical manifestations of scabies. _____

_____

Chapter **25** **The Child with Major Alterations in Tissue Integrity**

48. How should a scabicide lotion be applied to the skin? _____

_____

Atopic Dermatitis

49. The majority of children with atopic dermatitis develop _____ or _____.

50. What causes the intense pruritus associated with atopic dermatitis? _____

_____

51. Describe the appearance of the skin in childhood-onset eczema. _____

_____

52. List three interventions that can relieve itching for a child with atopic dermatitis.

    a. _____

    b. _____

    c. _____

Seborrheic Dermatitis

53. The most common form of seborrheic dermatitis is _____.

54. Name two clinical manifestations of seborrheic dermatitis.

    a. _____

    b. _____

55. Give two interventions used to treat cradle cap.

    a. _____

    b. _____

Contact Dermatitis

56. What is contact dermatitis? _____

57. Name three interventions that can relieve itching from contact dermatitis.

    a. _____

    b. _____

    c. _____

58. What initial interventions should be taken if a child is exposed to poison ivy? _____

_____

Answer as either true (T) or false (F).

59. _____ Diaper dermatitis is easier to prevent than to treat.

60. _____ The diaper area should be cleaned with water and mild soap after each voiding or bowel movement.

61. _____ Rubber pants should not be used because they hold in moisture and cause skin breakdown.

Acne Vulgaris

62. What parts of the skin are involved in acne vulgaris? _____

63. Develop an explanation of acne for a young adolescent. _____

_____

64. What should the nurse teach an adolescent about the following medications to prevent adverse effects?

    a. Tetracycline: _____

    b. Isotretinoin (Accutane): _____

65. What guidelines for daily skin care should be followed by the adolescent with acne?

_____

_____

Insect Bites or Stings

66. What precautions should be taken when a child is allergic to bee stings? _____

_____

_____

67. What intervention should be taken when a child gets a bee sting? _____

_____

68. Why should insect repellents containing diethyltoluamide (DEET) not be used on young children?

_____

Miscellaneous Skin Disorders

69. Describe the management of frostbite. _____

_____

70. What should children and parents know about preventing frostbite? _____

_____

71. Describe the best method of removing a tick. _____

_____

     Chapter **25** The Child with Major Alterations in Tissue Integrity

Match each skin disorder with its definition.

72. _____ Stevens-Johnson syndrome

73. _____ Molluscum contagiosum

74. _____ Psoriasis

75. _____ Warts

a. Viral infection of the skin and mucous membranes
b. Chronic inflammatory condition caused by rapid proliferation of keratinocytes
c. Skin infection caused by a human papilloma virus
d. Autoimmune disease that may be triggered by infections or medications

Burn Injuries

Match each description of burn injury with the corresponding level of burn depth. (Answers may be used more than once.)

76. _____ Blisters within minutes of burn injury

77. _____ Peels after 24 to 48 hours

78. _____ Has a mottled, waxy, white, dry surface

79. _____ White, cherry-red, or black appearance

a. Superficial
b. Partial thickness
c. Full thickness

Match each description of burn injury with the corresponding levels of severity. (Answers may be used more than once.)

80. _____ Partial-thickness burns of greater than 20% of total body surface area (TBSA)

81. _____ Full-thickness burn of less than 2% TBSA, not involving special areas

82. _____ Partial-thickness burns of 10% to 20% TBSA

83. _____ Burns of eyes, ears, face, hands, feet, perineum, or joints

a. Minor
b. Moderate
c. Major

84. What should the nurse teach parents about preventing sunburn in children? _____

_____

_____

85. List the three commonly used topical antimicrobial agents for burns.

a. _____

b. _____

c. _____

86. Define burn shock. _____

_____

87. Name four possible complications of an electrical injury.

a. _____

b. _____

c. _____

d. _____

88. The major cause of burn injuries to children younger than 3 years is _____.

SUGGESTED LEARNING ACTIVITIES

1. Develop a one-page instruction sheet for parents about any of the disorders presented in this chapter.

2. If possible, arrange an observational experience at a pediatric burn center.

3. What are your fears and concerns about caring for a child who has had a major burn injury?

STUDENT LEARNING APPLICATIONS

Enhance your learning by discussing your answers with other students.

The Child with Head Lice

Six-year-old Kelly was sent to the school nurse because her teacher noticed that she had been scratching her head for the past few days.

1. How should the school nurse check Kelly for head lice?

The examination of Kelly's head revealed nits throughout her hair. When the nurse called Kelly's mother to discuss the matter, her mother comments, "I wash Kelly's hair almost every day. She is a neat child. How could she get lice?"

2. How should the nurse respond to this comment?

3. What are the implications of this problem for the other children in the classroom? For other members of Kelly's family?

4. How should the nurse explain the treatment for head lice to the mother?

5. What measures should be taken in Kelly's classroom?

6. What can children be taught about preventing head lice?

The Child with a Burn Injury

Two-year-old Erica was burned when she pulled on a tablecloth and hot coffee spilled on her chest. On arrival at the emergency department, Erica is alert. Her vital signs are: temperature 98.4° F, heart rate 102 beats/min, respirations 24/min, blood pressure 86/54 mm Hg. A 5 × 10-cm area on her upper chest area is red, and four fluid-filled blisters are observed.

1. How would you classify the depth and severity of Erica's injury?

2. What would you expect to be included in Erica's treatment?

Chapter **25** **The Child with Major Alterations in Tissue Integrity**

Erica's parents are told that she can go home but that they will need to take care of her burned area until it heals.

3. What will you teach them about caring for a burn wound?

4. What concerns do you have about preventing burns in Erica's home?

5. How should you respond to Erica's mother when she asks you, "Will she have a scar?"

REVIEW QUESTIONS

Choose the best answer.

1. A child cut his hand a few days ago. Now the area is swollen and painful, and a red streak extends from it up to the forearm. These are signs of:
   a. impetigo.
   b. cellulitis.
   c. contact dermatitis.
   d. eczema.

2. Which medication is appropriate for the treatment of tinea capitis?
   a. Griseofulvin (Grisovin) orally for 6 weeks
   b. Lotrimin (Clotrimazole) cream to affected areas three times a day until lesions are healed
   c. Tinactin (Tolnaflate) spray twice per day to affected lesions
   d. Penicillin four times a day for 10 days

3. The stinger of a honeybee should be removed by:
   a. squeezing it out of the skin.
   b. using tweezers to lift it out.
   c. scraping it out horizontally.
   d. applying heat to draw out the stinger.

4. What should an adolescent female with severe acne know about isotretinoin (Accutane) before initiating treatment?
   a. Use of sunscreen will help to reduce the effect of photosensitivity from isotretinin (Accutane).
   b. Isotretinoin (Accutane) can cause menstrual irregularities.
   c. Isotretinoin (Accutane) is teratogenic if taken during pregnancy.
   d. Exposure to sunlight should be avoided while taking isotretinoin (Accutane).

5. What should the nurse teach parents about skin care for the child with atopic dermatitis?
   a. After bathing, apply moisturizing cream when the skin has been thoroughly dried.
   b. Avoid clothing made of cotton and polyester because these materials are irritating.
   c. Dress the child warmly at bedtime to prevent itching from coldness.
   d. Moisturizing creams can be applied whenever the skin looks dry.

6. Which action is appropriate for the prevention of diaper dermatitis?
   a. Apply medicated powder to perineum after each diaper change.
   b. Wash diaper area with a mild soap and water after each diaper change.
   c. Keep the diaper area open to air during rest periods.
   d. Change diapers at least every 4 hours.

7. Assessment of the skin of a child with diaper dermatitis is likely to reveal:
   a. keratosis.
   b. ecchymoses.
   c. lichenification.
   d. pruritus.

8. Assessment of a child with nits would reveal:
   a. very small black bugs jumping throughout the hair.
   b. white specks firmly attached to the hair shaft.
   c. small flakes resembling dandruff that are easily removed from the hair.
   d. clusters of nits at the crown of the head and front hairline.

9. The depth of a burn that appears red to pale ivory, with a moist surface and fluid-filled blisters, is most likely:
   a. superficial.
   b. superficial partial thickness.
   c. deep partial thickness.
   d. full thickness.

10. What is the first priority when initiating treatment on a child with a major burn injury?
    a. Fluid resuscitation
    b. Prevention of sepsis
    c. Airway assessment
    d. Correcting metabolic imbalances

11. What is the most common cause of burn injuries in children younger than 3 years of age?
    a. Flame
    b. Electrical
    c. Chemical
    d. Scald

12. Burn shock results from:
    a. hypovolemia.
    b. sepsis.
    c. toxins.
    d. metabolic acidosis.

13. Which statement made by a parent indicates correct understanding of how to manage seborrheic dermatitis on an infant's scalp?
    a. "I should massage the baby's head with oil after I wash her hair."
    b. "Use a soft toothbrush on the head when bathing to loosen the scales."
    c. "It is best to limit washing her hair so the scalp does not become dry."
    d. "I will apply moisturizing cream to the scalp several times a day."

14. What is the most appropriate response to a parent who asks for information about a salmon-patch birthmark?
    a. "This birthmark may appear darker when the baby is crying."
    b. "This is a permanent birthmark that often enlarges over time."
    c. "Surgical excision as soon as possible is the preferred treatment."
    d. "This common birthmark is associated with congenital syndromes."

15. The nurse is teaching a parent about the care of a 5-year-old child with contact dermatitis. Which statement made by the parent would indicate a correct understanding of the teaching?
    a. "I can allow my child to participate in all regular activities."
    b. "I should contact the physician if my child develops new lesions."
    c. "I can bathe my child in a tepid bath with an oatmeal-type bath product."
    d. "I should keep my child's room warm and use a humidifier at night."

16. The nurse is preparing to admit a 10-year-old with cellulitis of the leg with a high fever. Which interventions should the nurse include in the child's plan of care? *(Choose all that apply.)*
    a. Incision and drainage of the affected area may be necessary.
    b. Warm, moist soaks should be applied every 4 hours.
    c. Aspirin should be administered for fever or pain every 6 hours.
    d. IV antibiotic therapy should be administered at the same time each day.
    e. The affected leg should be dangled over the bedside every 12 hours.

Chapter **25** **The Child with Major Alterations in Tissue Integrity**

17. The nurse is teaching a 16-year-old with acne vulgaris about treatment for the condition. Which statement made by the adolescent would indicate a need for additional teaching?
    a. "I should scrub my face three times a day with an acne solution."
    b. "Acne cannot be cured but I can control the inflammation."
    c. "I should get regular rest mixed with appropriate exercise."
    d. "Acne treatment includes a topical medication with benzoyl peroxide in it."

26 The Child with a Musculoskeletal Alteration

HELPFUL HINT

Review the anatomy and physiology of the musculoskeletal system in an anatomy and physiology textbook.

STUDENT LEARNING EXERCISES

Definitions

Match each term with its definition.

1. _____ Avascular necrosis

2. _____ Dysplasia

3. _____ Callus

4. _____ Paresthesia

5. _____ Pseudarthrosis

6. _____ Reduction

7. _____ Subluxation

8. _____ Valgum

9. _____ Varum

a. Failure of the bones to fuse
b. Abnormal position of a bone in which it is bent away from the midline
c. Tissue damage resulting from inadequate blood supply to the area
d. Partial dislocation of a joint
e. Abnormal development of tissue
f. Abnormal position of a bone in which it is bent toward the midline
g. Repositioning of bone fragments into neutral alignment
h. Sensation of numbness and tingling
i. Tissue that joins fractured bone ends or repairs damaged bone

Recall the definition of the italicized term in each of the following. Then identify whether the statement is true (T) or false (F).

10. _____ Artificial limbs are called *orthoses*.

11. _____ *Callus* becomes hardened through osteoclastic activity.

12. _____ *Superior mesenteric artery syndrome* resembles intestinal obstruction.

13. _____ *Crepitus* results when the ends of a broken bone move.

14. _____ *Ankylosis* is a condition in which a joint is difficult to move.

15. _____ *Plantar flexion* involves bending the foot upward.

Review of the Musculoskeletal System

16. The sutures of the cranium fuse at approximately _____ months of age.

17. Why are fractures unusual in infants younger than 1 year of age? _____

_____

Chapter **26** **The Child with a Musculoskeletal Alteration**

Casts and Traction

18. Casts and traction are used to _____ a fracture.

19. Unless stated by the physician, the nurse should assume that traction is _____.

20. Skin traction is most effective in children who weigh less than _____ and who are younger than _____.

21. 90/90 femoral traction is _____ traction.

22. _____ is the most serious complication associated with skeletal traction.

23. List the five Ps of vascular impairment.

    a. _____

    b. _____

    c. _____

    d. _____

    e. _____

24. Identify two nursing responsibilities for a child in traction.

    a. _____

    b. _____

Limb Defects and Clubfoot

Answer as either true (T) or false (F).

25. _____ Clubfoot is readily apparent by clinical examination at birth.

26. _____ An infant's clubfoot cannot be manipulated into a neutral position.

27. _____ Nonsurgical management of clubfoot requires serial casting.

28. _____ Genu valgum is commonly referred to as "bowlegs."

29. _____ Children requiring casts for limb abnormalities are at risk for altered growth and development.

30. _____ Genu varum is a normal variation in toddlers.

31. _____ A child with webbed fingers has polydactyly.

Developmental Dysplasia of the Hip

32. What are the manifestations of developmental dysplasia of the hip in the following age-groups?

    a. Newborn/young infant: _____

    b. Older infant: _____

174

33. The Pavlik harness maintains the hip in which three positions? _____

_____

34. Improper positioning of an infant's hip in a Pavlik harness can interrupt the blood supply to the head of the femur, resulting in _____.

35. Information for parents about caring for their infant in a Pavlik harness would include:

a. _____.

b. _____

c. _____

d. _____

Legg-Calvé-Perthes Disease

Answer as either true (T) or false (F).

36. _____ The most common symptom of Legg-Calvé-Perthes disease (LCP) is persistent pain in the hip.

37. _____ LCP results in avascular necrosis of the femoral head.

38. _____ Surgical correction increases overall treatment time.

39. _____ In LCP, both hips are usually affected.

Slipped Capital Femoral Epiphysis

40. The typical adolescent with slipped capital femoral epiphysis (SCFE) is _____ average for height and weight.

41. What symptoms would prompt the nurse to suspect that an adolescent has SCFE? _____

_____

Fractures

42. A fractured bone in an infant warrants investigation to rule out _____.

43. A fracture to the epiphyseal plate of a bone can interfere with _____

_____.

44. Nursing assessment of a child with a traumatic fracture begins with _____

_____.

45. A systemic risk associated with fractures is _____.

46. Describe compartment syndrome. _____

_____

_____

Chapter **26** **The Child with a Musculoskeletal Alteration**

47. Proper healing of a fracture requires correct reduction and _____

48. Open reduction requires the surgical insertion of a(n) _____
    device.

Soft Tissue Injuries

Match each term with its definition.

49. _____ Sprain

50. _____ Strain

51. _____ Contusion

52. _____ Dislocation

a. Articulating surfaces of joint no longer in contact
b. Damage to soft tissue, muscle, or subcutaneous tissue
c. Excessive muscle stretch, resulting in tears and pulls
d. Stretched or torn ligaments

53. Control of _____ is essential with a soft tissue injury.

54. The nurse would assess the child with a soft tissue injury for _____ and

    _____ .

Osgood-Schlatter Disease

55. To what is Osgood-Schlatter disease thought to be related? _____

    _____

56. List three clinical manifestations of Osgood-Schlatter disease.

    a. _____.

    b. _____

    c. _____

Osteogenesis Imperfecta

57. Describe osteogenesis imperfecta. _____

    _____

58. Identify three clinical manifestations of osteogenesis imperfecta.

    a. _____.

    b. _____

    c. _____

Osteomyelitis

Answer as either true (T) or false (F)

59. _____ The most common causative agent of osteomyelitis in all ages is *Staphylococcus aureus*.

60. _____ Cellulitis can result in osteomyelitis.

176

61. _____ The manifestations of osteomyelitis are vague and nonspecific in older children.

62. _____ Children with osteomyelitis require complete bed rest.

63. Identify three nursing responsibilities for a child receiving antibiotics for osteomyelitis.

   a. _____.

   b. _____

   c. _____

Juvenile Arthritis

64. Briefly describe juvenile arthritis. _____

   _____

65. What is uveitis? _____

66. When are slow-acting antirheumatic drugs used? _____

   _____

67. A priority nursing diagnosis for a child with juvenile arthritis might be _____

   _____.

Muscular Dystrophies

68. Muscular dystrophies are a group of _____, _____ diseases that affect muscle cells of specific muscle groups.

69. What is the most common type of muscular dystrophy? _____

70. What is the most common cause of death resulting from muscular dystrophy? _____

   _____

Scoliosis, Kyphosis, and Lordosis

Answer as either true (T) or false (F).

71. _____ Idiopathic scoliosis is the predominant form of scoliosis.

72. _____ Uneven shoulder height is an indicator of scoliosis.

73. _____ For treatment of scoliosis, a brace is worn 22 to 23 hours per day.

74. _____ Spinal fusion is used to treat severe scoliosis.

SUGGESTED LEARNING ACTIVITIES

1. Spend some time with a school nurse performing scoliosis screenings. Report on the procedure, the reactions of the students, and the screening results to your class.

2. Observe in a newborn nursery. Observe the nurses' techniques for assessing skeletal abnormalities.

Chapter **26** **The Child with a Musculoskeletal Alteration**

STUDENT LEARNING APPLICATIONS

Enhance your learning by discussing your answers with other students.

Twelve-year-old Kai is admitted to the hospital with a fractured femur. He is in Russell traction, and he says to you, "I hate this thing! Why are you doing this to me?"

1. How would you explain to Kai about traction and why he needs it?

2. How would you address the "doing this to me" aspect of Kai's question?

3. How would you facilitate trust?

4. How would you enlist Kai's cooperation in maintaining proper alignment and in doing range-of-motion exercises and neurovascular assessments?

REVIEW QUESTIONS

Choose the best answer.

1. In which period is screening for idiopathic scoliosis done?
   a. Prenatally
   b. In the newborn period
   c. During the school-age years
   d. In middle adolescence

2. Which assessment finding would be suggestive of developmental dysplasia of the hip?
   a. Unable to flex leg and hip
   b. Crying when hip is palpated
   c. Asymmetry of gluteal folds
   d. Guarding of the affected leg

3. When developmental dysplasia of the hip is diagnosed:
   a. treatment is begun immediately.
   b. treatment is postponed until the child is able to bear weight.
   c. surgery is scheduled as soon as the child weighs 10 pounds.
   d. bilateral casting is done at 1 month of age.

4. A complication of uncorrected scoliosis would be:
   a. superior mesenteric artery syndrome.
   b. reduced respiratory function.
   c. fusion of the vertebrae.
   d. impaired physical mobility.

5. During an assessment, the nurse knows a child with lordosis may present with:
   a. a concave deformity and obesity.
   b. scoliosis and kyphosis.
   c. a convex deformity and pain in the lower back.
   d. unequal shoulder height and leg length discrepancy.

6. A newborn infant has been casted for a clubfoot. The nurse would teach parents about:
   a. assessing for genu varum.
   b. preventing pathologic fractures.
   c. frequent follow-up visits.
   d. preventing deformities in the hands.

7. A child has a closed fracture of the right radius, with slight ecchymosis below the elbow. The child rates her pain as either 9 or 10 on a 10-point scale. Her right hand is cooler than her left, and she cannot extend the fingers of her hand because they "burn." She probably has:
   a. compartment syndrome.
   b. epiphyseal injuries.
   c. early signs of an infection.
   d. paresthesia.

8. In taking the history of a child with juvenile arthritis, the nurse would probably discover that the child is taking:
   a. acetaminophen.
   b. aspirin.
   c. morphine.
   d. prednisone.

9. A male adolescent is diagnosed with Osgood-Schlatter disease. In taking a history the nurse is not surprised to find that he:
   a. is below the 20th percentile for height and weight.
   b. is a medal-winning swimmer.
   c. is on the football team.
   d. has a family history of arthritis.

10. A painful limp, pain in the knee and hip joints, and quadriceps muscle atrophy are clinical manifestations of:
    a. Legg-Calvé-Perthes disease.
    b. Osgood-Schlatter disease.
    c. Osteogenesis imperfecta.
    d. Duchenne muscular dystrophy.

11. An appropriate nursing intervention for a child's sprained ankle is:
    a. ice packs applied for 20 minutes.
    b. a warm compress for 30 minutes.
    c. position affected foot lower than the body.
    d. position affected foot higher than the heart.

12. What is the best way for the nurse to assess sensory function in a 6-year-old child with a lower leg cast?
    a. Ask "Do you feel this?" when pressing down on the little toe.
    b. Check capillary refill in the middle toe.
    c. Request the child to wiggle his toes.
    d. Ask "Which toe am I pinching?" when pinching the great toe.

13. When planning to discuss bracing for correction of scoliosis with a 13-year-old girl, the nurse would expect the girl's primary concern to be:
    a. discomfort and pain.
    b. risk for injury.
    c. fear of surgery.
    d. appearance.

14. A musculoskeletal condition that typically results in death in late adolescence is:
    a. osteogenesis imperfecta.
    b. Legg-Calvé-Perthes disease.
    c. Duchenne muscular dystrophy.
    d. juvenile arthritis.

15. A child with a fractured tibia and fibula had a plaster cast applied to the lower leg. Which statement made by the child's parent indicates a need for additional teaching about cast care?
    a. "I am going to lift the cast gently with my fingertips."
    b. "I should put ice on the cast for 24 to 48 hours."
    c. "The leg in the cast should be elevated on a pillow."
    d. "A fan blowing cool air will help the cast to dry."

16. The nurse is caring for a 7-year-old with osteomyelitis. Which clinical findings would the nurse expect to observe? *(Choose all that apply.)*
    a. Erythema and tenderness over the site
    b. Limited range of motion
    c. Elevated sedimentation rate
    d. Decreased C-reactive protein level
    e. Intermittent radiating pain

17. The nurse is teaching the parent of a 14-year-old newly diagnosed with juvenile idiopathic arthritis. Which statement by the parent would indicate a correct understanding of the teaching?
    a. "I should expect my child to move slowly in the evening."
    b. "I should administer NSAIDs to my child before breakfast."
    c. "My child should not receive the annual flu vaccine."
    d. "My child should have foods that are high in protein, fiber, and calcium."

18. Place in the correct sequence the steps for controlling swelling and reducing muscle damage of a soft tissue injury.
    a. Ice
    b. Compression
    c. Rest
    d. Elevation

27 The Child with an Endocrine or Metabolic Alteration

Refer to an anatomy and physiology textbook for a more extensive discussion of the endocrine system. It may also help to refer to Chapters 3 and 12 in your textbook.

STUDENT LEARNING EXERCISES

Definitions

Match each term with its definition.

1. _____ Hormone
2. _____ Gland
3. _____ Pituitary
4. _____ Euthyroid
5. _____ Glucagon
6. _____ Hyperglycemia
7. _____ Hypoglycemia
8. _____ Hypothalamus

a. An endocrine gland attached to the base of the brain that secretes numerous hormones
b. Chemical substance produced by one gland or tissue and transported by the blood to other tissues, where it causes a specific effect
c. Blood glucose levels below 70 mg/dL
d. Portion of the brain that secretes releasing factors
e. Organ or structure that secretes a substance to be used in some other part of the body
f. Normal thyroid function
g. In a non-diabetic person, fasting blood glucose level greater than or equal to 110 mg/dL
h. Counteracts the action of insulin

Review of the Endocrine System

Match each hormone with the pituitary lobe that produces it. (Pituitary lobes may be used more than once.)

9. _____ Oxytocin
10. _____ Adrenocorticotropic hormone
11. _____ Thyroid-stimulating hormone
12. _____ Luteinizing hormone
13. _____ Antidiuretic hormone
14. _____ Growth hormone
15. _____ Prolactin

a. Anterior pituitary lobe
b. Posterior pituitary lobe

Diagnostic Tests and Procedures

16. How are alterations in endocrine functioning usually diagnosed? _____

_____

17. Accurate measurement of _____ and _____ are essential when assessing a child for endocrine function.

Neonatal Hypoglycemia

18. Hypoglycemia in the neonate is defined as a plasma glucose concentration of less than _____.

19. The neonates who are most likely to have hypoglycemia are _____ infants and infants who are _____.

20. List five signs that indicate a neonate is hypoglycemic.

    a. _____

    b. _____

    c. _____

    d. _____

    e. _____

21. What is the intervention for a neonate who is hypoglycemic but asymptomatic? _____

    _____

    _____

22. What nursing assessments are indicated if a neonate is at increased risk for hypoglycemia?

    _____

    _____

    _____

23. What complication can occur when a neonate is receiving intravenous glucose? _____

    _____

    _____

Hypocalcemia

24. Neonatal hypocalcemia is defined as total serum calcium concentration of less than _____.

25. Why does neonatal hypocalcemia occur most often in infants of diabetic mothers? _____

    _____

    _____

Phenylketonuria and Inborn Errors of Metabolism

26. What is the genetic transmission pattern of phenylketonuria? _____

27. Phenylketonuria results in damage to which body system? _____

28. When should the neonate be screened for phenylketonuria? _____

29. What is the treatment of phenylketonuria? _____

_____

Answer as either true (T) or false (F).

30. _____ The child with galactosemia must be on a life-long, low-protein, limited amino acid diet.

31. _____ Maple syrup urine disease causes ketoacidosis 2 to 3 days after birth.

32. _____ Tay-Sachs disease can be treated through dietary modifications.

Congenital Adrenal Hyperplasia

33. In congenital adrenal hyperplasia, the adrenal gland is not able to manufacture _____but
    instead produces excess _____.

34. What finding in the newborn infant would raise suspicion of congenital adrenal hyperplasia? _____

_____

_____

35. The treatment of congenital adrenal hyperplasia involves life-long _____

_____.

Congenital and Acquired Hypothyroidism

Answer as either true (T) or false (F).

36. _____ Newborn screening for hypothyroidism should be done between 10 and 14 days of age.

37. _____ If untreated, congenital hypothyroidism can result in mental retardation.

38. _____ Treatment of congenital hypothyroidism requires life-long thyroid hormone replacement.

39. _____ The most common cause of acquired hypothyroidism in children is thyroiditis.

40. _____ A decreased thyroid-stimulating hormone level is the most sensitive indicator of primary hypothyroidism.

Chapter **27** **The Child with an Endocrine or Metabolic Alteration**

Match each disorder with its characteristic signs and symptoms. (Disorders may be used more than once.)

41. _____ Decreased activity

42. _____ Nervousness

43. _____ Increased appetite

44. _____ Weight gain

45. _____ Edema of face, hands, and eyes

46. _____ Cold intolerance

a. Hypothyroidism
b. Hyperthyroidism

Hyperthyroidism (Graves Disease)

47. The preferred treatment for a child with hyperthyroidism is _____.

48. The child receiving propylthiouracil must be monitored for which three adverse effects?

    a. _____

    b. _____

    c. _____

49. List two nursing diagnoses for a child with hyperthyroidism.

    a. _____

    b. _____

Diabetes Insipidus

50. Diabetes insipidus results when there is a deficiency of _____.

51. List the two classic manifestations of diabetes insipidus.

    a. _____

    b. _____

52. How is a water deprivation test diagnostic of diabetes insipidus? _____

_____

_____

53. What medication is used to treat diabetes insipidus? _____

54. How is this medication administered? _____

_____

Syndrome of Inappropriate Antidiuretic Hormone

55. What is the body's response to excessive antidiuretic hormone? _____

_____

56. In syndrome of inappropriate antidiuretic hormone:

    a. Urine output is _____.

    b. Urine specific gravity is _____.

    c. Serum sodium levels are _____.

    d. Fluid is _____.

57. The child with fluid overload is at risk for injury related to _____ caused by hyponatremia.

Precocious Puberty

58. Define *precocious puberty*. _____

59. What is a major consequence of precocious puberty? _____

60. The treatment for true precocious puberty is _____.

61. How does the therapy in question 60 work to inhibit precocious puberty? _____

_____

Growth Hormone Deficiency

Answer as either true (T) or false (F).

62. _____ A sign that a child may have a growth hormone deficiency is if his or her weight is less than the 5th percentile for age and sex.

63. _____ Delayed puberty is a manifestation of growth hormone deficiency.

64. _____ Stimulation testing is necessary to confirm a diagnosis of growth hormone deficiency.

65. _____ Growth hormone replacement is administered subcutaneously six or seven times per week.

Diabetes Mellitus

66. The primary source of energy for body cells is _____.

67. Glucose is stored in the liver and muscles in the form of _____.

68. The main function of insulin is _____.

69. What is the etiology of type 1 diabetes mellitus? _____

Identify the physiologic basis for the following signs and symptoms of type 1 diabetes mellitus.

70. Hyperglycemia: _____

71. Polyuria: _____

72. Excessive thirst: _____

73. Hunger: _____

74. Weight loss: _____

Match each sign or symptom with its cause. (Causes may be used more than once.)

75. _____ Tachycardia

76. _____ Fruity breath

77. _____ Kussmaul respirations

78. _____ Blurred vision

79. _____ Irritability

80. _____ Abdominal pain

    a. Adrenergic symptom of hypoglycemia
    b. Neuroglycopenic symptom of hypoglycemia
    c. Ketoacidosis
    d. Hyperglycemia

81. A fasting serum glucose level exceeding _____ and a random level exceeding _____ is indicative of type 1 diabetes mellitus.

82. Why is insulin administered parenterally? _____

83. What criteria must be met for an adolescent with type 1 diabetes mellitus to be considered for an insulin pump?

    a. _____

    b. _____

    c. _____

    d. _____

Answer as either true (T) or false (F).

84. _____ The child in the "honeymoon" phase requires increased insulin therapy to prevent hyperglycemia.

85. _____ The goal of insulin therapy is to assist the beta cells with insulin production.

86. _____ Oral hypoglycemic agents are not effective in the management of type 1 diabetes mellitus.

87. _____ Food intake should be balanced with insulin dosage.

88. _____ The family should adhere to a consistent schedule for meal times and amount of food intake.

89. _____ Exercise raises blood sugar levels.

90. _____ Exercise should be scheduled to coincide with insulin peak times.

91. _____ A 15- to 30-g carbohydrate snack can be eaten when the child is planning one hour of exercise.

92. List one task that a child in each of the following age groups can be expected to do in the management of type 1 diabetes mellitus.

    a. Toddler/preschooler: _____

    b. School-age child: _____

    c. Early adolescent: _____

    d. Middle/late adolescent: _____

93. What situations could result in hypoglycemia? _____

_____

94. What intervention for hypoglycemia should be taken if the child is unconscious? _____

_____

95. Identify the expected laboratory results for the child in diabetic ketoacidosis as low, normal, or elevated.

    a. Blood glucose: _____

    b. Urinary ketones: _____

    c. Arterial pH: _____

_____

    d. Serum potassium: _____

96. Why is rehydration the initial step in resolving diabetic ketoacidosis? _____

_____

97. Why would the child in diabetic ketoacidosis have Kussmaul respirations? _____

_____

98. What type of insulin and route of administration are used in the treatment of diabetic ketoacidosis?

_____

_____

Chapter **27** **The Child with an Endocrine or Metabolic Alteration**

99. What would the nurse teach parents about managing a child's type 1 diabetes mellitus during periods of minor illness?

_____

_____

Answer as either true (T) or false (F).

100. _____ Many children diagnosed with type 2 diabetes mellitus are overweight.

101. _____ In type 2 diabetes mellitus, the pancreas no longer produces insulin.

102. _____ Life-long insulin injections are required for the management of type 2 diabetes mellitus.

SUGGESTED LEARNING ACTIVITIES

1. Arrange to observe an outpatient endocrine clinic. Because many children with endocrine alterations are treated in outpatient settings, this would provide firsthand knowledge of pediatric endocrine alterations.

2. Develop a teaching plan for the parents of a newborn infant diagnosed with congenital hypothyroidism.

3. Review teaching materials for type 1 and type 2 diabetes mellitus used at your clinical site. Compare them with teaching materials at another site.

4. Talk with children who have type 1 and type 2 diabetes mellitus and their families about management and living with this chronic disease.

STUDENT LEARNING APPLICATIONS

Enhance your learning by discussing your answers with other students.

The Child with Type 1 Diabetes Mellitus

Lizzy is a 7-year-old who has been sent to the emergency department from the pediatrician's office for possible diabetic ketoacidosis. Her parents brought her to the pediatrician because she has had increased urination and abdominal pain. She has lost weight over the past few weeks. The emergency department nurse observes Lizzy breathing rapidly and deeply and notes that her breath has a fruity odor. Lizzy's blood glucose is 580 mg/dL. Her parents are shocked when they are told that Lizzy has diabetic ketoacidosis. Her father says, "We thought she might have a urinary tract infection."

1. Why might he have thought Lizzy had such an infection?

Her mother then comments, "My father developed diabetes a few years ago. Could that be why Lizzy has diabetes?"

2. How would you respond to the mother's question?

3. What is the basis for Lizzy's symptoms?

4. What interventions would you expect for Lizzy?

5. What would you expect Lizzy's insulin schedule to be?

Lizzy and her parents receive intensive teaching about type 1 diabetes mellitus management. She is placed on a schedule of three insulin injections per day. A few days later, her mother calls the nurse because Lizzy is pale, shaky, and diaphoretic.

6. What do you think is happening to Lizzy?

7. What action would you take?

Lizzy has been active in soccer and softball at her school, and she wants to continue to play.

8. What can Lizzy do to prevent problems during a game or practice?

The Child with Diabetes Insipidus

Danny is a 9-year-old boy who recently underwent removal of a craniopharyngioma. Last night he frequently requested drinks of water and his urine output was 1000 mL. His urine tested negative for glucose and his urine specific gravity was 1.003.

1. What do you suspect is the cause of Danny's symptoms?

2. What other assessments would you make when diabetes insipidus is suspected?

Danny's thirst and increased urination continue throughout the day. When Danny's mother is told that Danny's symptoms are being caused by diabetes insipidus, she reacts by saying, "He's been through so much already. Now something else."

3. How would you respond to Danny's mother?

Danny is started on desmopressin intranasally He asks, "How long will I have to take this stuff?"

4. How would you respond to Danny?

5. What would you teach Danny and his mother about desmopressin?

6. List nursing diagnoses and outcomes for this situation.

REVIEW QUESTIONS

Choose the best answer.

1. Which of these statements about congenital hypothyroidism is correct?
   a. Mental retardation caused by hypothyroidism is reversible with treatment.
   b. The most common cause of congenital hypothyroidism is thyroiditis.
   c. The child with congenital hypothyroidism requires life-long thyroid hormone replacement.
   d. Screening for this disorder is usually done between 3 and 6 months of age.

2. The child with precocious puberty is at risk for:
   a. altered reproductive ability.
   b. delayed development of secondary sex characteristics.
   c. short adult stature.
   d. endocrine tumors.

3. A clinical manifestation of growth hormone deficiency is:
   a. weight less than 5th percentile for age and sex.
   b. hyperglycemia.
   c. precocious puberty.
   d. height less than 5th percentile for age and sex.

Chapter **27**   **The Child with an Endocrine or Metabolic Alteration**

4. A nursing intervention for a child with syndrome of inappropriate antidiuretic hormone secretion is to:
   a. offer fluids frequently to increase fluid intake.
   b. explain the reason for restricting fluids.
   c. assist the child in selecting low sodium foods.
   d. assess the child for dehydration.

5. A nursing diagnosis appropriate for the child with diabetes insipidus is:
   a. Excess Fluid Volume related to decreased urine output.
   b. Deficient Fluid Volume related to abnormal fluid loss from polyuria.
   c. Risk for Injury from seizures related to hyponatremia.
   d. Risk for Injury from altered acid-base balance related to lack of insulin.

6. When performing a physical assessment on a child with hyperthyroidism, the nurse would be alert for:
   a. coarse hair.
   b. dry thick skin.
   c. cold intolerance.
   d. tremors.

7. The child with syndrome of inappropriate antidiuretic hormone would be assessed for signs of the electrolyte imbalance called:
   a. hyponatremia.
   b. hypernatremia.
   c. hypocalcemia.
   d. hypokalemia.

8. The etiology of type 1 diabetes mellitus is thought to be:
   a. viral.
   b. genetic.
   c. environmental.
   d. autoimmune.

9. A child received regular insulin subcutaneously at 8 AM. At what time is this child most likely to become hypoglycemic?
   a. Between 8 AM and 9 AM
   b. Between 10 AM and 11 AM
   c. Between noon and 2 PM
   d. Between 3 PM and 5 PM

10. Which of these situations could lead to hypoglycemia?
    a. Insufficient insulin
    b. Decreased exercise
    c. Missed meal
    d. Minor illness

11. An appropriate diabetes task for the preschool child would be to include:
    a. performing finger puncture for blood.
    b. choosing injection sites according to a rotation schedule.
    c. pushing the plunger on the syringe.
    d. identifying a phrase to describe hypoglycemia.

12. Sick day rules for the child with type 1 diabetes mellitus include:
    a. not giving insulin if the child is nauseated or vomiting.
    b. testing blood glucose levels at least twice a day.
    c. testing urine for ketones with each void.
    d. offering fluids with calories if the child is not eating.

13. One adrenergic sign of hypoglycemia is:
    a. blurred vision.
    b. clammy skin.
    c. irritability.
    d. increased respiratory rate.

14. If not properly balanced with insulin and diet, exercise can lead to:
    a. hypoglycemia.
    b. hyperglycemia.
    c. ketoacidosis.
    d. hypokalemia.

15. The best action for a child when he is hypoglycemic is to:
    a. drink 4 ounces of fruit juice.
    b. eat a chocolate bar.
    c. drink a can of diet soda.
    d. get some exercise.

16. What is the body's response to an inability to produce insulin?
    a. Glucose is transported into the cell at a rapid rate.
    b. The liver converts fats to ketones for energy.
    c. Carbohydrate metabolism is increased.
    d. Hypoglycemia occurs as glucose in insulin is stored in the liver as glycogen.

17. The nurse is preparing to admit a child with hypothyroidism. Which clinical manifestations would the nurse expect to observe? *(Choose all that apply.)*
    a. Dry, thick skin
    b. Course, dull hair
    c. Weight loss
    d. Exophthalmos
    e. Cold intolerance
    f. Irregular menses

18. The nurse is teaching the parent of a 12-year-old with type 2 diabetes mellitus. Which statement made by the parent would indicate a need for additional teaching?
    a. "I should encourage my child to eat foods that are reduced in saturated and *trans* fatty acids."
    b. "I should let my child exercise when he feels like it rather than set a schedule."
    c. "I should teach my child the benefits of carbohydrate counting to improve glycemic control."
    d. "I should have my child check his blood glucose levels two or three times per day."

19. What are signs and symptoms of ketoacidosis? *(Choose all that apply.)*
    a. Clammy skin
    b. Blurred vision
    c. Acetone breath
    d. Abdominal pain
    e. Dry mucous membranes
    f. Sudden weight gain

28 The Child with a Neurologic Alteration

HELPFUL HINT

Review the physiology of the nervous system in an anatomy and physiology textbook. Also refer to a pharmacology textbook for a more detailed discussion of anticonvulsant medications.

STUDENT LEARNING EXERCISES

Definitions

Match each term with its definition.

1. _____ Blood-brain barrier

2. _____ Cerebral herniation

3. _____ Cushing response

4. _____ Decerebrate posture

5. _____ Decorticate posture

6. _____ Monro-Kellie doctrine

7. _____ Myelinization

a. Abnormal flexion of the upper extremities and extension of the lower extremities
b. Formation of the proteolipid coating of nerves
c. Separation between brain tissue and blood
d. Shift of brain tissue sideways or downward, causing severe neurologic dysfunction
e. Abnormal extension of upper extremities with internal rotation of upper arms and wrists
f. Theory describing a compensatory mechanism of cranial contents that maintains steady volume and pressure
g. Late sign of increased intracranial pressure

Review of the Central Nervous System

8. Identify the week(s) during gestation when the following occur.

a. Neural tube closes: _____

b. First period of rapid brain cell growth: _____

c. Second period of rapid brain cell growth: _____

d. Myelin sheath begins to form: _____

9. Name the three main sections of the brain.

a. _____

b. _____

c. _____

10. What is the function of cerebrospinal fluid?

_____

Match each term with its description.

11. _____ Dura mater

12. _____ Tentorium

13. _____ Pia mater

14. _____ Axial skeleton

15. _____ Cerebrum

16. _____ Brainstem

a. Fills the upper portion of the skull
b. First layer of meninges
c. Contains the pons, medulla, midbrain, thalamus, and third ventricle
d. Tent-like structure separating cerebellum from occipital lobe
e. Innermost layer of meninges
f. Protects structures of the central nervous system

17. Describe the purpose of each of the following diagnostic tests.

   a. Computerized tomography (CT scan): _____

   _____

   b. Electroencephalography (EEG): _____

   _____

   c. Lumbar puncture: _____

   _____

   d. Magnetic resonance imaging (MRI): _____

   _____

   _____

18. Identify three nursing diagnoses that apply to children with disorders of the nervous system.

   a. _____ .

   b. _____

   c. _____

19. What is the rationale for maintaining the head of the bed at an angle between 30 and 45 degrees for a child with a neurologic disorder?

   _____

20. What positions should be avoided for a child who has a neurologic disorder? _____

   _____

21. Why might a child with a neurologic disorder have a nursing diagnosis of Imbalanced Nutrition: Less than Body Requirements?

_____

_____

Increased Intracranial Pressure

22. Identify two clinical manifestations of increased intracranial pressure for each of the following age-groups.

   a. Infants: _____

   b. Children: _____

23. Identify the following illustrations as decerebrate posturing or decorticate posturing.

   a. _____.

   b. _____

a

b

24. What three assessments are included in the Glasgow Coma Scale?

   a. _____.

   b. _____

   c. _____

Match each level of consciousness with its description.

25. _____ Confused

26. _____ Disoriented

27. _____ Lethargic

28. _____ Obtunded

29. _____ Stupor

30. _____ Coma

a. Person requires considerable stimulation to arouse
b. Ability to think clearly and rapidly is lost
c. Person awakens easily but exhibits limited responsiveness
d. Person is unable to recognize place or person
e. Vigorous stimulation produces no motor or verbal response
f. Person sleeps unless aroused

Answer as either true (T) or false (F).

31. _____ Changes in a child's normal behavior are important indicators of increased intracranial pressure.

32. _____ The pupils constrict as intracranial pressure increases.

33. _____ The progression from decerebrate to decorticate posturing indicates deterioration of the child's condition.

34. _____ The appearance of the Cushing reflex is an early sign of increased intracranial pressure.

Spina Bifida

35. Spina bifida results from _____.

36. Define the following terms.

   a. Meningocele: _____

   b. Myelomeningocele: _____

Answer as either true (T) or false (F).

37. _____ The degree of impairment is related to the level of the defect on the spinal cord.

38. _____ Folic acid deficiency in the mother has been linked to neural tube defects.

39. _____ A child with a myelomeningocele below S3 will have serious motor impairment.

40. _____ Prenatal screening involves measurement of maternal serum alpha-fetoprotein.

41. _____ Before surgery the neonate with a myelomeningocele is at risk for infection.

42. _____ Children with spina bifida are at high risk for development of a latex allergy.

Hydrocephalus

43. The treatment for hydrocephalus is _____

Match each clinical manifestation with the corresponding age group. (Age-groups may be used more than once.)

44. _____ Full, bulging anterior fontanel

45. _____ Nausea and vomiting that may be
projectile

46. _____ "Setting sun" eyes

47. _____ Shrill, high-pitched cry

48. _____ Widely separated cranial sutures

49. _____ Frontal headache in the morning
relieved by vomiting or sitting upright

50. _____ Seizures

a. Infant early sign
b. Infant late sign
c. Child early sign
d. Child late sign

Cerebral Palsy

Match each classification of cerebral palsy with its description.

51. _____ Spastic

52. _____ Ataxic

53. _____ Dyskinetic (athetoid)

a. Slow, writhing movements of all extremities
b. Increased deep tendon reflexes, hypertonia, flexion, and contractures
c. Loss of coordination, equilibrium, and kinesthetic sense

Answer as either true (T) or false (F).

54. _____ Almost all children with cerebral palsy will have some degree of mental retardation and other handicaps.

55. _____ In cerebral palsy the damage to the pyramidal motor system can occur in the prenatal, perinatal, or postnatal periods.

56. _____ A delay in motor development is a key indicator of cerebral palsy.

57. What type of equipment is included in bedside seizure precautions? _____

_____

_____

Head Injury

58. Name four common causes of head injuries in children.

a. _____ .

b. _____

c. _____

d. _____

59. What is included in the initial assessment of a child with a head injury? _____

_____

60. What guidelines should parents follow in determining when to notify the physician of a child's head injury?

_____

_____

61. What is *postconcussion syndrome?* _____

_____

Match each type of head injury with its description

62. _____ Contusion

63. _____ Concussion

64. _____ Closed head injury

65. _____ Epidural hemorrhage

66. _____ Subdural hemorrhage

a. Transient and reversible neuronal dysfunction with instantaneous loss of responsiveness
b. Accumulation of blood between the dura and skull
c. Petechial hemorrhages along the superficial aspects of the brain
d. Accumulation of blood between the dura and the cerebrum
e. Nonpenetrating injury to the head

Spinal Cord Injury

Answer as either true (T) or false (F).

67. _____ Immediately after a spinal cord injury at any level, flaccid paralysis of the limbs occur.

68. _____ A common cause of spinal cord injury in an infant is aggressive shaking.

69. _____ Most spinal cord injuries in children occur in the cervical spine.

70. _____ Before any attempt is made to move a child with a neck or spinal cord injury, the spine must be immobilized.

71. _____ After a spinal cord injury, the spinal cord is immobilized with the use of tongs or halo traction.

Seizure Disorders

Match each classification of seizure with its description.

72. _____ Tonic-clonic

73. _____ Atonic

74. _____ Myoclonic

75. _____ Absence

a. Sustained, generalized contraction of muscles followed by alternating contraction and relaxation of major muscle groups
b. Brief, random contractions of a muscle group
c. Brief episodes of altered consciousness characterized by a blank facial expression
d. Abrupt loss of postural tone, loss of consciousness, confusion, lethargy, and sleep

76. Differentiate between a seizure and epilepsy. _____

_____

_____

77. What are the pathophysiologic mechanisms of a seizure? _____

_____

78. Precipitating factors in febrile seizures are the _____ and _____ of temperature elevation.

79. What information should be elicited from a parent or caregiver when a child has a seizure?

_____

_____

80. List five nursing interventions to maintain a child's safety during a generalized tonic-clonic seizure.

a. _____.

b. _____

c. _____

d. _____

e. _____

81. What would a nurse teach parents about use of the anti-epileptic medication phenytoin (Dilantin)?

_____

_____

82. Define *status epilepticus.* _____

_____

Meningitis

83. What diagnostic test confirms that a child has meningitis? _____

84. What is meant by a positive Kernig sign? _____

_____

85. What is meant by a positive Brudzinski sign? _____

_____

86. How is acute bacterial meningitis treated? _____

_____

Answer as either true (T) or false (F).

87. _____ Symptoms of meningitis may be vague and nonspecific.

88. _____ The treatment of viral meningitis is symptomatic and supportive.

89. _____ There are no long-term sequelae associated with bacterial meningitis.

Guillain-Barré Syndrome

90. What is the most prominent feature of Guillain-Barré syndrome? _____

_____

91. The focus of nursing assessments for a child with Guillain-Barré syndrome would be the

_____ and _____ systems.

92. Identify three nursing diagnoses for a child with Guillain-Barré syndrome.

    a. _____.

    b. _____

    c. _____

Headaches

93. Identify five factors that are known to trigger the onset of a headache.

    a. _____.

    b. _____

    c. _____

    d. _____.

    e. _____

94. How does a migraine headache differ from a tension headache? _____

_____

_____

SUGGESTED LEARNING ACTIVITY

1. With use of the Glasgow Coma Scale, assess the neurologic status of several children.

Enhance your learning by discussing your answers with other students.

A father brings his 4-year-old daughter, Lisa, to the emergency department because she has had a seizure. He explains that she became unconscious, her body became rigid, and her back began arching and relaxing. Lisa has also had a headache, stiff neck, and fever for the past day.

1. What information in this situation is suggestive of meningitis?

2. What diagnostic study would confirm this diagnosis? What would you expect an analysis to reveal?

3. What other diagnostic study might be ordered for Lisa, given her history?

4. What additional information about Lisa's seizure should you gather from her father?

5. Lisa's father then asks, "What caused the seizure?" How would you respond?

6. As you are speaking with the father, Lisa begins to have a seizure like the one her father described.
   a. How would you classify this seizure?
   b. What nursing actions are indicated during a seizure?
   c. What would you document about the seizure?

7. What is the treatment for bacterial meningitis?

8. Lisa is admitted to the hospital. As her nurse, what assessments would you make?

REVIEW QUESTIONS

Choose the best answer.

1. During which week of gestation does the neural tube close?
   a. Fourth
   b. Eighth
   c. Sixteenth
   d. Twentieth

2. Which method is used to monitor brain growth?
   a. Cerebrospinal fluid analysis
   b. Head circumference measurement
   c. Electroencephalogram
   d. CT scan

3. Which manifestations would a nurse observe in a 4-month-old with increased intracranial pressure? *(Choose all that apply.)*
   a. Slurred speech
   b. Nausea and vomiting
   c. Papilledema
   d. Bulging fontanel
   e. Restlessness
   f. Setting-sun sign

4. What is a typical nursing intervention for a child with a head injury, who exhibits signs of the syndrome of inappropriate antidiuretic hormone secretion?
   a. Initiate seizure precautions.
   b. Monitor for dehydration.
   c. Restrict fluids.
   d. Assess for hypernatremia.

5. If a child awakens easily but exhibits limited responsiveness, his level of consciousness is described as:
   a. confused.
   b. disoriented.
   c. lethargic.
   d. stuporous.

6. Which element is not included in the Glasgow Coma Scale?
   a. Eye opening
   b. Motor response
   c. Verbal response
   d. Neurovascular status

7. Which change in vital signs is not associated with the Cushing reflex?
   a. Increased systolic pressure
   b. Decreased heart rate
   c. Increased temperature
   d. Irregular respiratory pattern

8. A newborn infant has a sac in the lumbosacral area containing spinal fluid, meninges, nerve roots, and the spinal cord. This condition is referred to as:
   a. myelomeningocele.
   b. meningocele.
   c. Arnold-Chiari malformation.
   d. spina bifida occulta.

9. Before surgery, the priority for care of a newborn infant with a myelomeningocele is:
   a. preventing infection.
   b. preserving urinary function.
   c. promoting nutrition.
   d. maximizing motor function.

10. An early sign of hydrocephalus in an infant is:
    a. "setting-sun" eyes.
    b. frontal bone enlargement.
    c. shrill, high-pitched cry.
    d. widely separated cranial sutures.

11. Which symptom suggests a problem with a ventriculoperitoneal shunt?
    a. Decreased level of consciousness
    b. Nausea
    c. Abdominal pain
    d. Paresthesia

12. Which type of cerebral palsy is characterized by increased deep tendon reflexes, hypertonia, and flexion of extremities?
    a. Spastic
    b. Ataxic
    c. Athetoid
    d. Rigid

13. An expected finding in an analysis of cerebrospinal fluid in the child with bacterial meningitis is:
    a. low protein.
    b. cloudy appearance.
    c. high glucose.
    d. increased red blood cells.

14. An appropriate nursing intervention during a tonic-clonic seizure is:
    a. restraining flailing extremities.
    b. placing padding between the teeth.
    c. observing the type of movements and the duration of the seizure.
    d. placing the child in a supine or prone position.

15. A parent describes his child as having a blank stare with eyelid twitching. This child is most likely having which type of seizure?
    a. Complex partial
    b. Atonic
    c. Myoclonic
    d. Absence

16. What is the first priority when a child has sustained a spinal cord injury?
    a. Assess motor function.
    b. Assess sensory function.
    c. Immobilize the spine.
    d. Measure vital signs.

17. Which statement about febrile seizures is true?
    a. Epilepsy will develop in the majority of children who have febrile seizures.
    b. Febrile seizures most commonly occur in children older than 5 years of age.
    c. Seizure activity occurs during a rise in temperature.
    d. A prolonged temperature elevation usually precedes the febrile seizure.

18. A child who sustained a head injury had loss of consciousness of less than 5 minutes and a Glasgow Coma Score of 14. This head injury would be classified as which severity of head injury?
    a. Severe
    b. Moderate
    c. Mild
    d. Minimal

19. The nurse is caring for an 11-year-old with increased intracranial pressure. Which interventions should be included in the child's plan of care? *(Choose all that apply.)*
    a. Monitor the child's pupil size and reactivity every hour.
    b. Place the child in the supine position with the neck flexed.
    c. Weigh the child daily at the same time on the same scale.
    d. Avoid clustering the child's care to ensure decreased stimulation.
    e. Reposition the child every 2 hours to asses for skin breakdown.
    f. Measure head circumference daily.

20. The nurse is teaching a parent of a 3-year-old who suffered a head injury. Which statement made by the parent indicates a correct understanding of the teaching?
    a. "My child may have a concussion but no further brain damage can occur."
    b. "I should expect my child to have a severe headache with vomiting."
    c. "My child may suffer from postconcussion syndrome and exhibit irritability if tired or stressed."
    d. "I should only contact the physician if my child has a seizure."

21. The nurse is teaching a 16-year-old with a seizure disorder about anti-epileptic medications. What information should the nurse include in the teaching?
    a. In most states a driver's license can be obtained if the adolescent has been on the anti-epileptic medications for 1 month.
    b. Birth control pills may be less effective for an adolescent while taking anti-epileptic medications.
    c. An adolescent can continue to play contact sports while taking anti-epileptic medications.
    d. Manic behavior may be seen with an adolescent when an anti-epileptic medication is started.

29 The Child and Family with Psychosocial Alterations

HELPFUL HINT

Review a psychiatric nursing textbook for additional information about psychosocial disorders and psychotropic medications.

STUDENT LEARNING EXERCISES

Definitions

Complete the following crossword puzzle.

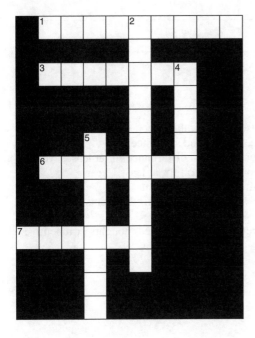

Across

1. Physical or psychological dependence on a substance even when it is known to impair cognitive or social functioning
3. Characterized by recurrent episodes of binge eating
6. Voluntary and intentional cessation of one's life
7. Statement or behavior that usually occurs before overt suicidal activity

Down

2. Presence of two different but interactive conditions existing simultaneously in a single individual
4. Non-accidental act of omission by a parent or caregiver
5. Exertion of extreme force or destructive action resulting in injury

Overview of Childhood Psychopathology

Answer as either true (T) or false (F).

8. _____ Cognitive development proceeds from abstract to concrete thinking.

9. _____ A significant factor affecting the impact of brain damage on the child is the maturational stage of the brain at the time the damage occurs.

10. State the rationale for performing each of the following diagnostic studies for psychosocial disorders in children and adolescents.

a. Urine tests: _____

b. Blood and serum tests: _____

c. Radiographs of the skull and long bones: _____

d. Measurement of subcutaneous tissue: _____

e. Genital and anal examinations: _____

Anxiety and Mood Disorders

Match each disorder with its description.

11. _____ Obsessive-compulsive disorder

12. _____ Dysthymic disorder

13. _____ Bipolar mood disorder

14. _____ Major depressive disorder

15. _____ Separation anxiety

16. _____ Posttraumatic stress disorder

a. Two-week episode of irritable mood with disturbances in sleep, appetite, energy, and self-esteem
b. Chronic fluctuating mood disturbance for at least 1 year
c. Irritable or depressed mood for at least 1 year
d. Anxiety felt after a terrifying event
e. Disabling fear about being away from parents or away from home
f. Manifests as repetitive uncontrolled thoughts or repetitive actions

Answer as either true (T) or false (F).

17. _____ Children with mood disorders have increased serotonin levels.

18. _____ Psychosocial disorders have been shown to have a genetic basis.

19. _____ A child or adolescent may have both anxiety and a mood disorder.

20. Which classification of medications is frequently prescribed for the treatment of anxiety and mood disorders?

_____

Suicide

21. Identify five manifestations that indicate a child is at risk for suicide.

a. _____

b. _____

c. _____

d. _____

e. _____

22. List three questions a nurse could ask an adolescent when he or she says that life is not worth living anymore.

a. _____

b. _____

c. _____

23. Describe the best approach for the nurse to take when an adolescent has expressed thoughts of suicide.

_____

_____

Answer as either true (T) or false (F).

24. _____ Poor self-concept is a significant factor in suicide.

25. _____ Screening children for depression in the school system is a poor suicide prevention strategy.

26. _____ Most suicide statements by adolescents can be ignored.

27. _____ Gay and lesbian adolescents are more likely to attempt suicide than their heterosexual peers.

Eating Disorders: Anorexia Nervosa and Bulimia Nervosa

28. Identify three distinguishing characteristics of anorexia nervosa.

a. _____

b. _____

c. _____

29. Identify three distinguishing characteristics of bulimia nervosa.

a. _____

b. _____

c. _____

Chapter **29** **The Child and Family with Psychosocial Alterations**

Answer as either true (T) or false (F).

30. _____ Adolescents with eating disorders usually have a family history of emotional disorders.

31. _____ Individuals with eating disorders often exhibit ritualistic tendencies about food preparation and food consumption.

32. _____ An adolescent with bulimia is at risk for tooth erosion.

33. _____ When assessing an adolescent with an eating disorder, it is best to use an unstructured format to elicit information.

Attention-Deficit Hyperactivity Disorder

34. Children with attention-deficit hyperactivity disorder (ADHD) have problems in what three areas?

a. _____

b. _____

c. _____

35. How is a diagnosis of ADHD established? _____

_____

36. The primary nursing intervention for the child with ADHD is: _____

_____

Answer as either true (T) or false (F).

37. _____ It may take several weeks to see the effects of stimulant medication on the behavior of a child with ADHD.

38. _____ Increased levels of norepinephrine in the brain have been associated with ADHD.

39. _____ ADHD affects boys more often than girls.

40. _____ Research indicates that food additives and sugars significantly aggravate behavior in children with ADHD.

41. _____ Children with ADHD tend to have fewer behavioral problems in chaotic environments.

Substance Abuse

42. What is a gateway substance? _____

43. List four behaviors that would alert the school nurse to a child's substance abuse.

a. _____

b. _____

c. _____

d. _____

Answer as either true (T) or false (F).

44. _____ The treatment of substance abuse includes individual, group, and family therapy.

45. _____ In a substance abuse treatment facility, the nurse's primary responsibility is to stabilize the patient's psychological status.

46. _____ It is important for the patient and family to identify and develop social support systems.

Infants with Neonatal Abstinence Syndrome

47. Fill in the manifestations of withdrawal for an infant born addicted to narcotics.

W: _____

I: _____

T: _____

H: _____

D: _____

R: _____

A: _____

W: _____

A: _____

L: _____

48. Identify three nursing interventions that are appropriate to decrease environmental stimuli for a newborn infant undergoing withdrawal.

a. _____

b. _____

c. _____

Childhood Physical and Emotional Abuse and Neglect

49. Identify three common characteristics of the abusive family.

a. _____

b. _____

c. _____

50. Define *shaken baby syndrome.* _____

_____

Chapter **29** **The Child and Family with Psychosocial Alterations**

51. Define *Munchausen syndrome by proxy.* _____

_____

52. Give two possible nursing interventions for the following nursing diagnosis: Impaired Parenting related to lack of knowledge.

a. _____

b. _____

Answer as either true (T) or false (F).

53. _____ The underlying problem for most forms of child abuse is family dysfunction.

54. _____ In most cases the child is abused by a nonfamily member.

55. _____ The most frequent and severe physical abuse occurs in children younger than 4 years of age.

SUGGESTED LEARNING ACTIVITIES

1. Perform a mental status examination on a school-age child or an adolescent. Document your findings. Use the box "Mental Status Examination of Children" in this chapter as a guideline.

2. Complete the following table on the clinical manifestations of various forms of child abuse.

Type of Abuse	Physical Indicators	Behavioral Indicators
Physical abuse		
Physical neglect		
Emotional abuse		
Sexual abuse		

STUDENT LEARNING APPLICATIONS

Enhance your learning by discussing your answers with other students.

Alex is a fifth grader with attention-deficit hyperactivity disorder who began taking methylphenidate (Ritalin) three times a day at the beginning of the school year. Alex is supposed to go to the school nurse's office at lunchtime for his second dose of the day. Alex's cooperation with coming for his medication has been inconsistent. He told the school nurse that he just forgets to come.

1. Why do you think Alex has not been cooperative with coming for his medication?

2. If you were the school nurse, what strategies might you use to help Alex remember to come for his medication every day?

3. What assessments would you make for a child receiving methylphenidate?

Alex's teacher remarks that he is a different child now that he is taking methylphenidate.

4. Why would this medication make such a difference in a child's behavior?

5. Why should Alex take methylphenidate after eating lunch instead of before lunch?

REVIEW QUESTIONS

Choose the best answer.

1. Parents explain that their child has been irritable for the past month. The child has much less energy than usual and her grades have declined. This child meets the criteria for:
   a. dysthymic disorder.
   b. cyclothymic disorder.
   c. school phobia.
   d. major depressive disorder.

2. One of the most significant factors that contribute to teen suicide is:
   a. poor self-concept.
   b. anxiety.
   c. gender.
   d. introverted personality.

3. An adolescent tells the school nurse that he has thought about killing himself. An appropriate response to the adolescent would be:
   a. "I am going to call your parents about this."
   b. "I have the number of a suicide hotline."
   c. "How do you feel right now?"
   d. "Why would you even think about killing yourself?"

4. Which is *not* a manifestation of anorexia nervosa?
   a. Recurring episodes of binge eating
   b. Secondary amenorrhea
   c. Extreme fear of obesity
   d. Thin extremities with muscle wasting

5. The nurse might expect a child with attention-deficit hyperactivity disorder to be:
   a. a gifted student who is bored with school subjects.
   b. easily distracted by internal and external stimuli.
   c. able to complete one activity before moving to the next project.
   d. ritualistic about activities of daily living.

Chapter **29** **The Child and Family with Psychosocial Alterations**

6. Which family characteristic would put an adolescent at the most risk for substance abuse?
   a. Family practices an authoritarian parenting style.
   b. Family participates in school and community projects.
   c. Open communication among family members is encouraged.
   d. One parent has chronic physical and mental health problems.

7. An adolescent who uses drugs regularly and exhibits a physical dependence on the drug is considered to be in the phase of:
   a. experimentation.
   b. early drug use.
   c. true drug addiction.
   d. severe drug addiction.

8. A child has been coming to school early and staying late and is seen stealing food from the cafeteria. These behaviors are suggestive of:
   a. physical abuse.
   b. physical neglect.
   c. emotional abuse.
   d. sexual abuse.

9. The nurse is caring for a 15-year-old who is exhibiting signs of major depressive disorder. Which clinical manifestations would the nurse expect to observe. *(Choose all that apply.)*
   a. Angry outbursts
   b. Loss of interest in usual activities
   c. Chronic nightmares
   d. Decreased anxiety
   e. Irritability

10. The nurse is conducting a seminar for a group of adolescents about commonly abused drugs and their effects. Which statement made by an adolescent would indicate a correct understanding of the teaching?
    a. "Cocaine may cause distorted perceptions with hallucinations."
    b. "Amphetamines cause heightened awareness of surroundings."
    c. "Marijuana may cause a chronic cough and wheezing."
    d. "Opiates cause euphoria and elation with impaired judgment."

30 The Child with a Developmental Disability

Review growth and development of all age-groups in Chapters 4 through 8 of your textbook.

STUDENT LEARNING EXERCISES

Definitions

Match each term with its definition.

1. _____ Intelligence

2. _____ Pervasive developmental disorders

3. _____ Functional age

4. _____ Comorbidity

a. Occurrence of two or more disorders in an individual
b. Disorders involving impairment in several areas of development
c. Capacity of a child to learn, think, and solve problems
d. Age equivalent at which a child is able to perform specific self-care or relational tasks

5. Children with cognitive deficits have impairments in measured _____ and

_____ behavior.

Terminology

6. What criteria must be present for a diagnosis of mental retardation?

   a. _____

   b. _____

   c. _____

7. Identify four components of a developmental disability.

   a. _____

   b. _____

   c. _____

   d. _____

8. How did the Education for All Handicapped Children Act (Public Law 94-142) affect children with cognitive impairments?

   _____

   _____

9. What is an individualized education plan? _____

_____

Cognitive Impairment

10. Identify two reasons for the relationship between developmental disabilities and child abuse.

   a. _____

   b. _____

11. What is the cardinal sign of cognitive impairment?

   _____

12. Name the two most common genetic disorders in which cognitive impairment is a central feature.

   a. _____

   b. _____

Answer as either true (T) or false (F).

13. _____ There appears to be a strong association between a child's early neurodevelopmental functioning and later intellectual ability.

14. _____ Safety is a concern for cognitively impaired children.

15. _____ Disruptive behavior disorders or other psychiatric disorders often coexist with cognitive impairment.

16. _____ The diagnosis of mental retardation is most often made during the neonatal period.

17. _____ Therapeutic management for children with cognitive impairments largely depends on community and educational resources.

18. Identify three nursing diagnoses for the family of a child with a severe cognitive impairment.

   a. _____

   b. _____

   c. _____

Down Syndrome

19. The most common type of living experience for a child with Down syndrome is to be reared

   _____.

20. Down syndrome is generally diagnosed at birth as a result of the infant's _____.

Chapter **30** **The Child with a Developmental Disability**

21. List four areas the nurse should assess when caring for the child with Down syndrome.

a. _____

b. _____

c. _____

d. _____

Answer as either true (T) or false (F).

22. _____ Down syndrome is the most common genetic disorder causing moderate to severe mental retardation.

23. _____ Most children with Down syndrome are born to women older than 35.

24. _____ In almost all instances, Down syndrome is the result of translocation of chromosome 21 to chromosome 15.

25. _____ When a child with Down syndrome is cared for in the hospital, it is important to keep the environment and schedule as close to the child's usual environment and routines as possible.

Fragile X Syndrome

Answer as either true (T) or false (F).

26. _____ Fragile X syndrome is the most common inherited cause of mental retardation.

27. _____ Children with fragile X syndrome have no distinctive physical features.

28. _____ Fragile X syndrome is three times more common in girls than boys.

Fetal Alcohol Syndrome

29. What facial characteristics are associated with fetal alcohol syndrome? _____

_____

30. The infant with fetal alcohol syndrome is likely to have permanent _____

and _____ sequelae.

Answer as either true (T) or false (F).

31. _____ The use of alcohol during pregnancy is not totally necessary for a diagnosis of fetal alcohol syndrome.

Autism

32. Autism is classified as a _____.

33. List four developmental areas in which qualitative impairment is seen in children with autism.

a. _____

b. _____

c. _____

d. _____

213

34. What is the primary characteristic of autism? _____

Answer as either true (T) or false (F).

35. _____ Family child-rearing practices and parental personalities are the basis of the development of autism.

36. _____ The incidence of autism is equal in males and females.

37. _____ DNA testing is the definitive method of diagnosing autism.

38. _____ Autism usually becomes apparent after 3 years of age.

Match each disorder with its characteristic clinical manifestations. Disorders may be used more than once.

39. _____ Alzheimer-type dementia in adulthood

40. _____ Marked distress over minor changes in environment

41. _____ Protruding tongue, low-set ears

42. _____ Marked lack of awareness of feelings of others

43. _____ Flat feet, lax ankles, and hyperextensible fingers

44. _____ Possible presence of other medical conditions

45. _____ Prominent ears and long, narrow face

46. _____ Smooth philtrum and thin upper lip

a. Down syndrome
b. Fragile X syndrome
c. Autism
d. Fetal alcohol syndrome

Failure to Thrive

47. What is the most commonly observed risk factor for nonorganic failure to thrive? _____

_____

48. Identify the physical indicators of failure to thrive. _____

_____

49. Identify the behavioral indicators of failure to thrive. _____

_____

50. Identify interventions to increase caloric intake when feeding the child with failure to thrive.

_____

Answer as either true (T) or false (F).

51. _____ Increasing calorie intake is the first medical treatment initiated for a child with failure to thrive.

52. _____ Brain growth and development can be affected by undernutrition in the first 2 years of life.

SUGGESTED LEARNING ACTIVITIES

1. Talk with parents of a child with a cognitive deficit. Discover what support systems they are using both within the family and in the community.

2. Spend some time in a local law library and research educational laws related to children with cognitive deficits. Report your findings to the class.

3. Interview an occupational therapist or other member of the multidisciplinary team. Discuss early intervention programs for the child with a cognitive deficit.

STUDENT LEARNING APPLICATIONS

Enhance your learning by discussing your answers with other students.

Jean Marie, a 4-year-old preschooler, is an outpatient at the pediatric clinic. Routine pediatric follow-up data indicate that she has consistently achieved developmental milestones, but she reaches them much later than children of the same chronologic age. Her physical appearance is normal. Jean Marie's weight and height are within the normal range for a child her age. She has been healthy throughout childhood, with only minor illnesses.

1. What further assessment data would you need for Jean Marie?

2. What types of assessment would you do with her family?

3. Identify potential community resources that you could use for Jean Marie and her family at this stage of evaluation.

4. What would be your preliminary nursing diagnoses and interventions for Jean Marie?

REVIEW QUESTIONS

Choose the best answer.

1. Which of the following is a clinical manifestation of Down syndrome?
   a. Extremely soft and smooth skin
   b. Hypertonicity of large muscles
   c. Long, narrow face with large ears
   d. Single transverse palmar crease

2. The best method of detecting mental retardation at an early age is:
   a. neuropsychologic testing.
   b. analysis of results of an IQ test for cognitive abilities.
   c. developmental assessment at well-child care.
   d. radiographic evaluation of the brain.

3. The child with fragile X syndrome will exhibit:
   a. frustration with a change in routine.
   b. impairment in the rate of physical, social, and language skills.
   c. abnormal ways of relating to people.
   d. gaze avoidance, hand flapping, and abnormal speech patterns.

Chapter **30** **The Child with a Developmental Disability**

4. Which question asked during a hospital admission assessment best indicates that the nurse understands the needs of a child with Down syndrome?
   a. "Can you go over her daily routine with me?"
   b. "Does she require a special diet?"
   c. "Does she sleep through the night?"
   d. "Is she toilet trained?"

5. Injuries are less common among children with cognitive deficits during:
   a. infancy.
   b. toddlerhood.
   c. preschool age.
   d. adolescence.

6. The nurse assessing a child with autism would expect which findings?
   a. Hyperkinetic behavior, poor coordination, and cognitive deficits
   b. Absent or delayed speech and abnormal ways of relating to people
   c. A history of periods of remission and relapse
   d. Onset of the disorder during pubescence or adolescence

7. The goal for a child with a cognitive deficit is to:
   a. find an appropriate facility to meet the long-term needs of the child.
   b. maximize the child's skill potential and provide safe, nurturing care in a supportive family.
   c. use community resources to support the family through stressful periods.
   d. assist the child to live within his limitations.

8. In developing a plan of care for an infant with fetal alcohol syndrome, the nurse would anticipate parents to report difficulty in the infant's:
   a. feeding.
   b. mobility.
   c. speech.
   d. elimination.

9. What is the most appropriate response to a parent who asks the nurse, "What caused my child to have autism?"
   a. "The condition is passed from mother to sons on one of the X chromosomes."
   b. "It is likely that alcohol or drugs during pregnancy are the cause of your child's autism."
   c. "The exact cause is not known, but it is believed to be caused by structural abnormalities in the brain."
   d. "Late maternal age resulting in chromosomal alterations is thought to be associated with autism."

10. An acquired cause of cognitive impairment in children is:
    a. drug addiction.
    b. Down syndrome.
    c. lead poisoning.
    d. hypothyroidism.

11. A 9-month-old infant hospitalized with a diagnosis of nonorganic failure to thrive most likely:
    a. has intense stranger anxiety.
    b. cries constantly unless held by the mother.
    c. is extremely watchful of everyone in the room.
    d. is receptive to being held by the nurse.

12. Which guideline is appropriate for feeding a toddler who has not been gaining weight?
    a. Feed the child first; then allow him to attempt to feed himself.
    b. Serve different foods every day for variety.
    c. Give the child tasty junk food to increase calorie consumption.
    d. Try to keep meal and snack times the same each day.

13. Which conditions are causes of intellectual disabilities in children? *(Choose all that apply.)*
    a. Postmaturity
    b. Galactosemia
    c. Hyperbilirubinemia
    d. Congenital rubella
    e. Neonatal asphyxia

14. The nurse is conducting an in-service on the differential diagnosis of autism, intellectual disability and schizophrenia. What information should the nurse include in the in-service?
    a. Schizophrenia has an onset during pubescence or adolescence.
    b. Autism can be treated with medications.
    c. Intellectual disabilities have an increase occurrence of seizures.
    d. Autism demonstrates a flat skill profile.

Chapter **30** **The Child with a Developmental Disability**

31 | The Child with a Sensory Alteration

HELPFUL HINT

Review vision, hearing, and language development in Chapters 4 through 8 of your textbook. Also refer to Chapter 9 for an overview of screening techniques.

STUDENT LEARNING EXERCISES

Definitions

Complete the following crossword puzzle.

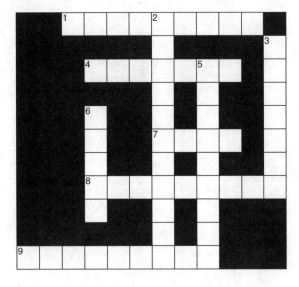

Across

1. Involuntary eye movements that make eyes appear to be darting back and forth
4. Hearing loss resulting from damage to the conduction system between the brain-stem and the cerebral cortex
7. Hearing loss characterized by the failure to hear 26 to 40 dB
8. Eyes turn away from the midline
9. _____ neonatorum

Down

2. Abnormal curvature of the cornea or the lens
3. Hemorrhage or sanguinous exudate in the anterior chamber of the eye
5. Reduced visual acuity not correctable by refractive means
6. Combination of conductive and sensorineural hearing loss

Review of the Eye and the Ear

Match each part of the eye or ear with its description.

10. _____ Eustachian tube

11. _____ Malleus, incus, and stapes

12. _____ Cochlea

13. _____ Tympanic membrane

14. _____ Retina

15. _____ Iris

16. _____ Cornea

17. _____ Macula

18. _____ Sclera

a. Small, snail-shaped chamber in the inner ear
b. Clear area located in the front of the eye
c. Structure that separates the outer ear from the middle ear
d. Inner area of the eye containing rods and cones
e. Structure that contains the greatest concentration of nerve endings in the eye
f. Structure that connects the middle ear with the nasopharynx
g. Bones of the middle ear
h. Colored muscular ring located behind the cornea
i. White outer covering of the eye

19. The critical period of eye development is _____ days' gestation.

20. The critical period for ear development is _____ weeks' gestation.

21. Binocularity is established by _____.

Speech Development

22. Babbling begins at _____ months.

23. Adequate _____ is essential for speech development.

Disorders of the Eye

Match each disorder with its description.

24. _____ Refractive error

25. _____ Strabismus

26. _____ Color blindness

27. _____ Glaucoma

28. _____ Cataract

29. _____ Conjunctivitis

30. _____ Orbital cellulitis

31. _____ Corneal abrasion

32. _____ Hyphema

a. Infection of the soft tissues surrounding the orbit
b. Misalignment of eyes resulting from lack of coordination of the extraocular muscles
c. Disorder resulting from a scraping of the lens
d. Alteration in the path of light rays through the eye
e. Inflammation of the clear membranous lining of the eyelid and sclera
f. Disorder caused by increased intraocular pressure
g. Hemorrhage resulting from a blow to the eye
h. Inability to distinguish among colors within certain groups
i. Opacity of the lens

33. The nurse plays an important role in the _____ and _____ of eye problems.

34. A primary concern for color blindness is _____.

35. How can a parent recognize a blocked lacrimal duct in an infant? _____

_____

36. What information would the nurse give a parent about the technique for lacrimal massage?

_____

_____

37. Define *legal blindness*. _____

38. What behaviors would suggest that a child has a refractive error? _____

_____

39. The nurse can assess visual acuity in a cooperative child as early as _____.

40. What complication can develop if amblyopia is not treated early? _____

_____

41. Why is eye patching used to treat amblyopia? _____

_____

42. What assessment findings would lead the nurse to suspect that a child has strabismus? _____

_____

43. What are the clinical signs of glaucoma? _____

_____

44. The preferred treatment for glaucoma in children is _____.

45. What signs of increased intraocular pressure must a child be monitored for postoperatively after eye surgery?

_____

_____

46. How should the nurse position the infant after cataract surgery? _____

_____

47. Identify four signs and symptoms of conjunctivitis.

    a. _____

    b. _____

    c. _____

    d. _____

48. What causes conjunctivitis in the first 24 hours of life? _____

    _____

49. What infection control measures should be used when a child has conjunctivitis? _____

    _____

    _____

50. Identify four nursing responsibilities for a child with orbital cellulitis.

    a. _____

    b. _____

    c. _____

    d. _____

51. A safety measure to prevent corneal abrasions and other eye injuries is _____

    _____.

52. What is the rationale for bed rest and eye patching in the treatment of hyphema? _____

    _____

53. What assessments should the nurse make when caring for a child with hyphema? _____

    _____

54. How should an eye be irrigated if it was splashed with a chemical? _____

    _____

Answer as either true (T) or false (F).

55. _____ Corneal ulceration may be a sign of underlying systemic disease.

56. _____ Amblyopia can be corrected at any time during childhood and adolescence.

57. _____ A blocked lacrimal duct is usually opened surgically before 1 year of age.

58. _____ Strabismus is a normal finding up to 3 months of age.

59. _____ The child should be able to decide how long to wear the eye patch each day.

60. _____ If detected early color blindness can be corrected.

61. _____ A chemical burn of the eyes should be irrigated immediately with water or saline solution.

62. _____ Of all sports activities, baseball and basketball are associated with the highest percentage of eye injuries.

Hearing Loss in Children

Match each type of hearing loss with its description.

63. _____ Central

64. _____ Conductive

65. _____ Mixed

66. _____ Sensorineural

a. Combination of conductive and sensorineural loss
b. Result of damage to the conduction system between the auditory nervous system and cerebral cortex
c. Result of damage or malformation of structures of the inner ear or auditory nerve
d. Sound prevented from progressing across the middle ear

67. Identify five risk factors that indicate a need for a neonate to have hearing screening.

   a. _____

   b. _____

   c. _____

   d. _____

   e. _____

68. The two hearing screening tests used to identify infants with hearing deficits are a(n)

   _____ and a(n) _____.

69. Name four guidelines for working with a hearing-impaired child.

   a. _____

   b. _____

   c. _____

   d. _____

Answer as either true (T) or false (F).

70. _____ The treatment for hearing loss depends on the type of loss.

71. _____ Sensorineural hearing loss is usually reversible.

72. _____ The recommended treatment for sensorineural hearing loss is a hearing aid.

73. _____ Deaf infants babble later than hearing infants.

74. _____ A child with recurrent otitis media with effusion lasting longer than 3 months should be evaluated for conductive hearing loss.

75. _____ All infants should have a hearing screening in their first month of life.

Language Disorders

Identify when the following milestones typically occur.

76. _____ Speaks first words

77. _____ Speaks first sentences

78. _____ Has a vocabulary of at least 50 words

79. Expressive language disorders affect which three areas of speech?

   a. _____

   b. _____

   c. _____

80. Identify three guidelines for parents on being effective role models in the area of speech.

   a. _____

   b. _____

   c. _____

Answer as either true (T) or false (F).

81. _____ Girls have more rapid language development than boys until 3 years of age.

82. _____ There is strong evidence linking early talking with greater intelligence.

83. _____ Children with a receptive language disorder are unable to understand the spoken word.

84. _____ Parents should begin reading to their child during infancy.

SUGGESTED LEARNING ACTIVITY

1. Observe a pediatric ophthalmologist, audiologist, or speech therapist. What techniques do these professionals use to assess infants and children for sensory disorders? What are the most common disorders that they encounter in their practices?

Enhance your learning by discussing your answers with other students.

Ten-year-old Jamie is developmentally delayed and blind. He was admitted to the hospital during the night for vomiting and abdominal pain. At the moment, he is moaning in pain. His IV is infiltrated, and he needs to have another IV line placed. Jamie's parents are not present.

1. What do you think Jamie's fears might be at this time? How would you address each of these fears?

2. Write down how you would explain to Jamie the procedure of placing an IV. What factors are you considering as you do this? What makes explaining this procedure difficult?

3. You learn that Jamie is going to the operating room for an appendectomy. How might preparing him for surgery differ from preparing a sighted child?

REVIEW QUESTIONS

Choose the best answer.

1. At what age does 20/20 vision normally develop?
   a. 4 years
   b. 5 years
   c. 7 years
   d. 8 years

2. Which of the following is a normal finding when assessing a 5-year-old's vision?
   a. Hyperopia
   b. Myopia
   c. Astigmatism
   d. Strabismus

3. Which are clinical signs of glaucoma? *(Choose all that apply.)*
   a. Blepharospasm
   b. Increased tearing
   c. Headache
   d. Light sensitivity
   e. Conjuctivitis

4. Which statement made by an adolescent indicates the need for additional teaching about eye care after conjunctivitis?
   a. "I threw out all of my eye shadow and bought new products."
   b. "I waited a week before I put my old contacts back in."
   c. "I change my mascara at least every 3 months."
   d. "I bought new eye liner so I wouldn't get pink eye again."

5. The nurse determines that a parent understands the correct technique for lacrimal massage when the parent says:
   a. "Massage from the inner eye down to the nasal bone."
   b. "Press gently in a circular motion."
   c. "Massage from the lacrimal duct upward."
   d. "Press inward on the lacrimal duct."

6. The nurse would explain the immediate intervention for a chemical burn to the eyes is to:
   a. flush with water and saline solution.
   b. apply antibiotic ointment.
   c. patch the affected eye.
   d. instill mydriatic drops to constrict the pupil.

7. During a hearing assessment, a child failed to hear a sound greater than 50 decibels. This hearing loss is considered to be:
   a. mild.
   b. moderate.
   c. severe.
   d. profound.

8. A cause of conductive hearing loss is:
   a. ototoxic medications.
   b. exposure to loud noises.
   c. otitis media.
   d. brain tumors.

9. What is an appropriate intervention to use when working with a child who has a hearing impairment?
   a. Maintain a soft background noise.
   b. Talk extremely slowly.
   c. Speak louder than usual.
   d. Use visual aids to assist your communication.

10. The nurse recognizes a delay in language development is suggested by:
    a. babbling at 6 months.
    b. saying three words at 18 months.
    c. having a vocabulary of 50 words at 2½ years.
    d. beginning to use two-word sentences at 3 years.

11. Which is *not* an expressive language disorder?
    a. Difficulty with fluency
    b. Difficulty with articulation
    c. Problem with pitch and articulation
    d. Problem with comprehending the spoken word

12. What information would the nurse include in discharge instructions for a child with hyphema?
    a. The affected eye should be patched every night for 2 weeks.
    b. The child can return to normal activities after discharge.
    c. Sports should be permanently avoided because of risk of re-injury.
    d. An eye shield must be worn at all times for several weeks.

13. A child tells the school nurse that he cannot see the words on the chalkboard. The nurse recognizes this finding as a sign of which eye disorder?
    a. Myopia
    b. Hyperopia
    c. Astigmatism
    d. Strabismus

14. The nurse is teaching the parent of a 6-year-old about eye patching after eye correction surgery. Which statement would indicate a need for additional teaching?
    a. "My child should continue to wear eyeglasses as normal."
    b. "My child can place the patch over a portion of the eye to prevent sweating."
    c. "I understand that the patching will not harm my child's stronger eye."
    d. "I should allow my child to decorate an extra patch and alternate wearing them."

15. The nurse is teaching a group of new nurses about different types of hearing loss. What information should the nurse include? *(Choose all that apply.)*
    a. Sensorineural hearing loss can be the result of damage to the auditory nerve.
    b. Central hearing loss is a combination of conductive and sensorineural conditions.
    c. Conductive hearing loss is often temporary and reversible.
    d. Central hearing loss may cause difficulty in differentiation of sounds and auditory memory.
    e. Conductive hearing loss progresses from inflammation of the inner ear to the outer ear.

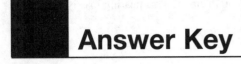

Answer Key

CHAPTER 1
Introduction to Nursing Care of Children

Student Learning Exercises

1. d
2. g
3. f
4. b
5. e
6. a
7. c
8. F
9. T
10. F
11. T
12. T
13. T
14. T
15. The efforts of ACCH have resulted in an increased awareness about the psychological and emotional effects of hospitalization during childhood. Hospital policies and health care services have changed, including 24-hour parental visitation, sibling visitation policies, child life programs in hospitals, shorter hospital stays, same-day surgery, and home care services.
16. A comprehensive, nationwide health promotion and disease prevention agenda.
17. Diagnosis-related grouping is a method of classifying related medical diagnoses on the basis of the amount of resources that are generally required by the client.
18. Case management is a practice model that identifies specific clients and manages their care collaboratively to ensure optimal outcomes through access to the best available resources.
19. Clinical pathways are standardized interdisciplinary plans devised for clients with specific health problems.
20. Medicaid and State Children's Health Insurance Programs (SCHIP).
21. WIC provides supplemental food supplies to low-income women who are pregnant or breastfeeding and to their children up to 5 years of age.
22. EPSDT provides comprehensive health care to Medicaid recipients from birth to 21 years of age.
23. PL 99–457 provides financial incentives to states to establish early intervention services for infants and toddlers with, or at risk for, developmental disabilities.
24. Healthy Start is an initiative to reduce infant deaths in communities with disproportionately high infant mortality rates.

25. T
26. T
27. F
28. T
29. c
30. a
31. d
32. b
33. F
34. T
35. T
36. Duty; breach of duty; damage; proximate cause
37. Client's competence to consent; full disclosure of information; client's understanding of information; client's voluntary consent
38. T
39. T
40. T
41. T
42. F
43. Care provider, teacher, collaborator, researcher, child and family advocate, manager of care
44. Nurse practitioners are advanced practice nurses who work according to protocols. They provide care for specific groups of clients in a variety of settings. Nurse practitioners may collaborate with a physician or work independently. Clinical nurse specialists are registered nurses who, through study and supervised practice at the graduate level, have become expert in the care of children and families. Clinical nurse specialists do not provide primary care. Four major sub roles have been identified for clinical nurse specialists: expert practitioner, educator, researcher, and consultant.
45. Clinics and physician offices; home health agencies; schools; rehabilitation centers; summer camps and day care centers; hospice or respite programs; psychiatric centers
46. e
47. b
48. c
49. a
50. d

Review Questions

1. c
2. b
3. c
4. a
5. a
6. c
7. c
8. b, d, e

CHAPTER 2
Family-Centered Nursing Care

Student Learning Exercises

1. e
2. a
3. d
4. c
5. f
6. b
7. The traditional nuclear family structure accounts for about 24.6% of all households in the United States. There is a growing number of nontraditional families, including single-parent families, blended families, adoptive families, unmarried couples with children, and multi-generational families. Most two-parent families are now dual-income families.
8. Single-parent, blended; adoptive; multigenerational; same sex partner; commune
9. Open communication; accurate perceptions about the nature and degree of the conflict; constructive efforts to resolve the conflict
10. E
11. I
12. I
13. E
14. I
15. F
16. F
17. T
18. T
19. T
20. F
21. T
22. T
23. F
24. F
25. T
26. Authoritarian; authoritative; permissive
27. F
28. F
29. T
30. F
31. **Easy:** even-tempered, predictable, regular in habits, and react positively to new stimuli.
    Difficult: highly active, irritable, moody, irregular in habits, adapt slowly to new

stimuli, and express intense negative emotions
    Slow-to-warm-up: inactive, moody, moderately irregular in habits, adapt slowly to new stimuli, and express mildly negative emotions
32. Discipline is a system of teaching and nurturing that prepares children to achieve competence, self-control, self-direction, and caring for others.
33. Positive, supportive, and loving relationship between parent(s) and child; use of positive reinforcement strategies to increase desired behaviors; using "time-out" or other alternatives that restrict undesired activity.
34. Redirection involves distracting the child by substituting an alternative activity or an object for the problematic one.
35. Time-out is a method of discipline that removes the attention given to a child who is misbehaving. The child is placed in a non-stimulating environment for a period of time, usually one minute per year of age.
36. Decrease in misbehavior is only short term; children learn that violence is acceptable; children become accustomed to pain, so parents may feel that more severe punishment is needed; parents may feel rage and lose control, causing harm to the child.
37. Behavior modification is a discipline technique that rewards positive behavior and ignores negative behavior.
38. F
39. F
40. T
41. T

Review Questions

1. c
2. a
3. a
4. c
5. b
6. c
7. a
8. c
9. a, b, e
10. c

CHAPTER 3
Communicating with Children and Families

Student Learning Exercises

1. c
2. f
3. e
4. d
5. a
6. b
7. T
8. F
9. T
10. F
11. F
12. T
13. F
14. T
15. F
16. Family-centered care emphasizes that the family is intricately involved in the care of the child. Health care professionals and families become partners in the care of the child. Family-centered care recognizes that the family has a right to participate in planning, implementing, and evaluating the child's plan of care.
17. Include all family members; encourage families to write down their questions; remain nonjudgmental; give families both verbal and nonverbal messages that convey openness and availability; respect and encourage feedback from families; avoid assumptions about core family beliefs and values; respect family diversity.
18. The nurse could establish rapport with families by conveying genuine respect and concern during the first encounter.
19. Understand the parents' perspectives; determine a common goal and stay focused on it; seek win-win solutions; listen actively; openly express your feelings; avoid blaming; summarize the decision.
20. As demographics change in the United States, nurses face the challenge of providing culturally competent care. Culture influences a family's values and beliefs and

communication style, methods of decision making, and other behaviors related to health care practices. Conflict may arise because of cultural differences.

21. Buying gifts for certain children; giving out a home phone number; competing with other staff for the child/family's affections; inviting child/family to social gatherings; accepting invitations to family gatherings; visiting child/family during off-duty time; revealing personal information; loaning money; making decisions for the family about the child's care.
22. T
23. F
24. F
25. F
26. Something along the lines of "I am going to take off the old bandage and put on a new one."
27. Something along the lines of "I am going to take you to a different room now. You can stay in this room while you are at the hospital."
28. Something along the lines of "I am going to give you medicine through a small needle."
29. Something along the lines of "I am going to measure your temperature" or "I am going to listen to your heart beating with my stethoscope."
30. Assess the child's self-help skills; orient child to surroundings; encourage parents to stay with child; keep furniture and objects in same places; explain sounds that child may hear; identify yourself when entering room; explain all procedures; keep call light in same place; allow child to handle equipment.
31. Assess the child's self-help skills; identify the family's method of communicating and adopt it; encourage parents to stay with the child; learn the child's sign language; develop a communication board; make sure hearing aids work; enter room cautiously and touch the child gently before speaking; face the child when

speaking; do not shout or exaggerate speech; use play to communicate and demonstrate procedures; have another person stand in front of the child if a procedure requires standing behind the child.

32. Assume the child can see, hear, and comprehend something in what is said; use a friendly tone of voice; address the child when entering and leaving the room; gently touch the child when saying his or her name; speak softly and slowly; do not talk as if the child were not there; explain all procedures as they are being done; talk to the child about activities and objects in the room; allow adequate time for child to respond to simple questions; ascertain child's ability to respond to simple questions; be attentive for signs and gestures that indicate likes or dislikes; document techniques that work.

Review Questions

1. b
2. b
3. d
4. b
5. a
6. d
7. c
8. a, c, e

CHAPTER 4
Health Promotion for the Developing Child

Student Learning Exercises

1. d
2. f
3. b
4. g
5. c
6. e
7. h
8. a
9. c
10. b
11. a
12. developmentally appropriate to meet the child's needs
13. growth
14. maturation
15. Development

16. learning
17. delays
18. a. school age, b. toddlerhood, c. adolescence, d. infancy, e. preschool age, f. newborn
19. Height; weight; head circumference
20. 6 months, 1 year
21. Head circumference
22. 20, 32
23. d
24. a
25. c
26. b
27. infancy, adolescence
28. Critical period refers to a block of time when children are able to master specific developmental tasks.
29. T
30. F
31. T
32. F
33. T
34. c
35. b
36. a
37. d
38. oral
39. phallic
40. genital
41. anal
42. latency
43. mistrust
44. Autonomy
45. Initiative
46. inferiority
47. Identity
48. b
49. a
50. c
51. cognitive
52. understand speech
53. produce meaningful speech
54. Crying
55. Heredity is the transmission of genetic characteristics from parent to child.
56. Assess for abnormalities; refer families to genetic counseling; act as advocates; support positive coping; provide education
57. genes, chromosomes
58. alleles
59. Autosomes
60. karyotype
61. e
62. h
63. b

64. g
65. a
66. j
67. i
68. k
69. d
70. f
71. c
72. It allows for comparison with statistical norms; it trends the child's growth pattern; it allows for early detection of abnormal growth patterns.
73. Observation; interview; physical examination; interactions with child and family; standardized assessment tools
74. Gross motor; fine motor; personal-social; language
75. T
76. F
77. T
78. F
79. Anticipatory guidance is basic information about normal growth and development given to parents as the child approaches a new developmental stage.
80. What does your child like to do at home? Describe your child's typical day. Can your child throw a ball, ride a tricycle, climb? Can your child draw pictures and color them? How effective is your child's use of language?
81. Those tasks done to amuse oneself that have behavioral, social, or psychomotor rewards
82. functional or sensorimotor play
83. represent concerns needing to be addressed
84. rules
85. e
86. c
87. b
88. d
89. a
90. T
91. F
92. F
93. T
94. T
95. F
96. c
97. e
98. a
99. b

100. d
101. Infants need sufficient calories to support rapid growth
102. 25%–35%
103. Hospitalization is already very stressful; the child does not need the added stress of unfamiliar foods.
104. 24-hour dietary recall; food frequency questionnaire; food diary
105. Unintentional injuries

Review Questions

1. b
2. a
3. c
4. a, b, c
5. d
6. c
7. b
8. b
9. d
10. d
11. d
12. c
13. d
14. c
15. d
16. a, d, e, f
17. c, a, b, d

CHAPTER 5
Health Promotion for the Infant

Student Learning Exercises

1. e
2. i
3. a
4. b
5. h
6. f
7. k
8. d
9. j
10. g
11. c
12. 8–9 months
13. 4–5 months
14. 4–5 months
15. 3 months
16. 6–7 months
17. 10–12 months
18. 6–7 months
19. 6–7 months
20. 1–2 months
21. 4–5 months
22. 8–9 months
23. 10–12 months

24. 1–2 months
25. 6–7 months
26. They have tiny, collapsible air passages and immature immune systems.
27. decreases; increases
28. Breast milk
29. 6–9 months
30. fluid and electrolyte imbalances
31. d
32. c
33. a
34. b
35. F
36. F
37. T
38. T
39. T
40. F
41. F
42. When infants' needs are ignored or not met adequately and consistently, they perceive the environment as unsafe and develop a sense of mistrust.
43. By mutually satisfying interactions between parent and infant. Parents adapt to their child through nurturing and by meeting the infant's needs.
44. At this age, infants recognize their caregivers and can distinguish them from strangers.
45. 3
46. immunologic; digestibility
47. Mothers who use illegal and certain prescription and over-the-counter drugs; mothers with tuberculosis; mothers with HIV infection
48. drinking from a cup
49. vitamin C
50. F
51. F
52. F
53. T
54. T
55. Holding them; speaking or humming softly to them; stroking them; massaging them; centering or swaddling them
56. Taking them on car rides; placing them in swings; walking with them; leaving them alone to "settle down" for no longer than 15 minutes
57. 120° ?
58. crawl

59. hot dogs; hard candy; grapes; peanuts; raisins; chewing gum

60. Infants should sleep in a crib with a firm mattress (not in the parents' bed). No toys or loose bedding should be in the crib. Avoid overheating and exposing the infant to environmental smoke. Offer the infant a pacifier at nap and bed time.

Review Questions

1. c
2. b
3. b
4. c
5. d
6. c
7. a
8. a
9. b
10. a
11. a
12. b, c
13. a, b, d, e
14. d

CHAPTER 6
Health Promotion during Early Childhood

Student Learning Exercises

1. i
2. d
3. f
4. n
5. k
6. b
7. m
8. e
9. h
10. a
11. j
12. l
13. g
14. c
15. 5
16. 2–3
17. 3
18. T
19. P
20. P
21. T
22. T
23. T
24. P
25. P
26. T
27. P

28. T
29. P
30. P
31. a
32. d
33. e
34. b
35. c
36. F
37. T
38. F
39. F
40. F
41. About 6 months after the first tooth appears.
42. They provide a sense of security and safety and decrease anxiety associated with increasing independence; they also provide them with a sense of control.
43. Nightmares awaken the child; night terrors do not wake the child and cannot be recalled.
44. discipline; limit setting
45. Time out; time in; using diversion; offering restricted choices
46. Never leave a child unattended in the tub; never leave buckets of water unattended; keep toilet lids closed.
47. To prevent injury from shoulder harnesses and lap belts by properly aligning seat belt.
48. Stop. Cover face with hands. Drop to the ground. Roll until the flames are out.
49. Keep guns unloaded, with trigger locks in place, locked in metal cabinets that are inaccessible to all children.
50. Teach children what constitutes appropriate touch; teach them to always tell another adult if someone touches them inappropriately, even if they are threatened; teach them to *keep telling* adults until the inappropriate behavior stops.
51. They will be less negative and more eager to please parents.
52. Limit stress; anticipate fatigue; prevent hunger; offer choices; be consistent; avoid overprotection
53. Before delivery, enroll the older child in sibling preparation classes. After delivery, encourage visitors and family to pay attention to the older

sibling; plan uninterrupted private time with the older child.
54. Focus on the ideas the child is expressing; do not complete words or sentences; avoid putting pressure on the child to communicate.

Review Questions

1. a
2. c
3. b
4. d
5. a
6. d
7. b
8. c
9. c
10. a
11. a, b, c
12. c
13. b, d, e

CHAPTER 7
Health Promotion for the School-Age Child

Student Learning Exercises

1. e
2. b
3. a
4. d
5. c
6. F
7. T
8. F
9. F
10. F
11. Active play increases coordination, refines motor skills, serves as a foundation for physical fitness as an adult, improves cardiovascular fitness, and increases strength and flexibility.
12. Children have higher metabolic rates.
13. actions
14. weight; volume
15. Cognitively, they are able to arrange things in logical order and are able to recall similarities and differences.
16. Their eustachian tubes have grown.
17. Children develop a sense of industry by learning to do new things and by learning to do them well.

18. As children learn to do things well, they become more confident and feel good about themselves. If they are unsuccessful, they lose confidence and develop a sense of inferiority.

19. Children learn that friendship is more than just being together. They begin to share problems and give each other emotional support. They develop a sense of loyalty.

20. a. Child obeys to avoid punishment; b. child obeys to avoid disapproval or to please others; c. child obeys out of respect for authority.

21. a. act; b. expectations; c. rewards, punishments

22. a. 6; b. 2.5; c. 1.5; d. 5; e. 3

23. 12; 9–10

24. Parents can foster a sense of responsibility in their children by making children accountable for their actions and by allowing them to experience their consequences.

25. Positively reinforce for effort; encourage self-discipline and good study habits; ensure adequate sleep; communicate with and support teachers

26. Nurses can act as advocates by knowing laws related to self-care children and by working to develop expanded after-school programs in their communities.

27. Children with separation anxiety feel distress whenever they are separated from their parents. Children with school phobia are only distressed at school.

Review Questions

1. b
2. d
3. c
4. a
5. b
6. b
7. c, e, f
8. d
9. c
10. b
11. a, d, e

CHAPTER 8
Health Promotion for the Adolescent

Student Learning Exercises

1. e
2. d
3. i
4. b
5. f
6. j
7. c
8. a
9. h
10. k
11. g
12. menstruation
13. peak height velocity (PHV)
14. breast buds (thelarche)
15. gynecomastia
16. Tanner staging or sexual maturity rating (SMR)
17. testicular enlargement
18. estrogen; testosterone
19. Assure confidentiality; be patient; remain nonjudgmental; assume nothing; use open-ended questions; encourage problem solving; be an advocate; do not side with adolescent against parents
20. A transition period granted to teens as they are experimenting with new roles and are not yet ready to make permanent commitments.
21. They provide safety for teens to experiment with new roles and they offer validation.
22. early
23. early
24. late
25. middle
26. middle
27. late
28. early; middle
29. middle
30. T
31. F
32. T
33. F
34. T
35. T
36. T
37. 46.8

Review Questions

1. d
2. a
3. d

4. c
5. c
6. a, b, c
7. d
8. b
9. b
10. b, c, e

CHAPTER 9
Physical Assessment of Children

Student Learning Exercises

1. g
2. d
3. i
4. l
5. j
6. a
7. m
8. e
9. h
10. k
11. c
12. f
13. b
14. T
15. T
16. F
17. T
18. T
19. T
20. indirect
21. fingertips
22. back of the hand
23. dull
24. bell
25. b
26. a
27. c
28. T
29. T
30. F
31. T
32. T
33. Use a measuring board or a tape measure with the child lying down.
34. It provides some indication of nutritional status and may detect tumor growth or an abnormal rate of development.
35. balanced
36. nipple line
37. muscle mass; fat
38. BMI = 22 (120.5 × 703/3844)
39. a. age, sex; b. horizontal; c. vertical; d. intersect; e. percentile
40. vitiligo

231

41. abdomen; upper arm
42. alopecia; hirsutism
43. hair
44. 1 to 2
45. V; VII
46. allergies
47. notch between the nose and upper lip
48. Ask the child to stick out the tongue as though licking a lollipop.
49. X
50. b
51. e
52. d
53. a
54. f
55. c
56. F
57. T
58. F
59. T
60. F
61. T
62. F
63. Adolescent girls should start performing breast self-examinations when they have reached menarche.
64. Auscultation follows inspection so that auscultation is not affected by percussion and palpation.
65. At a site away from the tenderness, place hand perpendicular to the abdomen, press down slowly, then lift hand.
66. Explain procedures, be honest and direct, and use a matter-of-fact approach.
67. Adolescent males are taught to do testicular examinations to screen for testicular cancer, which has a high incidence in young men.
68. T
69. F
70. T
71. F
72. T
73. T
74. T
75. T
76. F

Review Questions

1. d
2. c
3. b
4. a

5. b
6. d
7. d
8. a
9. b
10. c
11. c, b, d, a
12. d, b, c, a
13. b, d, e, f
14. c

CHAPTER 10
Emergency Care of the Child

Student Learning Exercises

1. b
2. d
3. h
4. c
5. e
6. g
7. a
8. f
9. Communicate an attitude of calm confidence; establish a trusting relationship with the child and family; try to avoid separating the child and parents; designate one staff member as caretaker of the child and liaison to the parents; tell the truth; provide incentives and rewards; and assess the child's unspoken thoughts and feelings.
10. Encourage the family members to move to a quiet place; encourage them to talk about their feelings as well as the facts; use reflective statements; avoid defensiveness, explanation, or justification of your own or others' behaviors; speak in simple sentences; set limits; help family to identify specific concerns and use their own effective coping strategies.
11. e
12. b
13. f
14. c
15. a
16. d
17. c
18. b
19. e
20. a
21. d
22. fear; anxiety

23. that the child will die
24. The triage nurse performs the initial observation in the emergency setting and decides the level of care needed for the child.
25. Respiratory rate and effort; skin color; response to the environment
26. A: airway; B: breathing; C: circulation; D: disability: neurologic assessment; E: exposure
27. T
28. T
29. F
30. T
31. T
32. F: full set of vital signs; G: give comfort measures/assess for pain; H: history and head-to-toe assessment; I: inspection/isolation
33. The correct order for measuring vital signs is respiratory rate, pulse, temperature, blood pressure.
34. S: signs and symptoms; A: allergies; M: medications taken, immunization history; P: prior illness or injuries; L: last meal, eating habits; E: events leading up to this illness or injury
35. Complete blood cell count with differential serum electrolytes, and urinalysis.
36. All medication dosages and fluid amounts are calculated according to the child's weight in kilograms.
37. Shock; respiratory failure
38. 20 per minute; 3–5
39. Perform the Heimlich maneuver.
40. CPR
41. A blind finger sweep is not performed because of the risk of forcing the object further down into the airway.
42. Place infant in downward-slanting position and administer five back blows, alternating with five chest thrusts.
43. brachial artery; carotid artery
44. 100 compressions per minute
45. five
46. H
47. C
48. D
49. D
50. C

51. C
52. H
53. F
54. T
55. F
56. F
57. T
58. T
59. T
60. F
61. T
62. Assess and manage life-threatening injuries.
63. Assessment and management of airway, breathing, circulation, and disability (neurologic assessment).
64. Assess for pain, inspect and document any and all signs of injury by performing a head-to-toe assessment, and obtain a history of the injury.
65. Motor vehicle: Was child wearing a seat belt or sitting in a child's car safety seat? What type of seat belt? What was the speed of the vehicle? With what did the vehicle collide? At what point on the motor vehicle was the location of impact? Where was the victim seated in the vehicle? How much damage was done to the vehicle?
Fall: How far did the child fall? How did the child land? On what type of ground did the child land? Did any objects "break" the child's fall? Penetrating injury: How long and wide was the blade of the knife? How far away was the gun when it was fired? What type of gun was used? What was the caliber of the gun?
66. Indicators: History inconsistent with physical findings; activity leading to the trauma inconsistent with the child's age and condition; delay in seeking treatment for the trauma; history of other emergency visits
Physical findings: Bruises and fractures in various stages of healing; injuries that are unusual for children; patterns of injury indicating that a specific object caused the injury
67. Continuous assessment of the child's respiratory, circulatory, and neurologic status

68. oral ingestion
69. Removal of dermal and ocular toxins; diluting the toxic substance; administering activated charcoal; giving antidote for the specific toxic substance
70. It does not completely remove the toxin; vomiting is uncomfortable for the child; it may interfere with subsequent interventions; it can be misused by others in the household (e.g., bulimic adolescents).
71. What substance was ingested? How much was ingested? What was the approximate time of ingestion? Has the child's condition changed from the time of ingestion? What treatment was administered at home?
72. Bite marks that look like fangs; burning at the site; ecchymosis and erythema; pain or numbness; edema
73. Wound irrigation and debridement; tetanus prophylaxis if not current; antibiotics if there is a high probability of infection; ice packs and elevation for pain
74. hypoxia
75. The diving reflex is stimulated when the face is submerged in cold water. Blood is shunted away from the periphery increasing blood flow to the brain and heart.
76. Respiratory system
77. Hope; privacy; comfort; contact person to provide them with updates and information
78. move the child to a cool place and start additional cooling measures.
79. Move the child to a cool place; start additional cooling measures such as loosening/removing wet clothes and applying cool, dry clothes. Offer oral fluids if there is no vomiting or alteration in mental status.
80. Hot, dry, red skin; change in level of consciousness or coma; rapid, weak pulse; rapid, shallow breathing; elevated core body temperature (>105° F)
81. F
82. T
83. F

Review Questions

1. c
2. c
3. d
4. b
5. b
6. c
7. d
8. d
9. a
10. c, d, e
11. c
12. a
13. c
14. c
15. a, c, d, e
16. b

CHAPTER 11
The Ill Child in the Hospital and Other Care Settings

Student Learning Exercises

1. e
2. d
3. f
4. c
5. a
6. b
7. Hospital, which can include 24-hour observation; emergency hospitalization; outpatient/day facilities; medical-surgical units; intensive care units; rehabilitative care; school-based clinics; community clinics; home care
8. T
9. T
10. F
11. F
12. T
13. T
14. T
15. T
16. Child's age; cognitive development; preparation; coping skills; culture; previous experiences with the health care system; parents' reactions to the illness
17. infant; toddler
18. Protest: Child is agitated, resists caregivers, cries, and is inconsolable.
Despair: Child is hopeless, quiet, withdrawn, and apathetic.
Detachment: Child may ignore parents but is interested in environment, plays, and seems to form relationships with caregivers and other children.

19. The nurse needs to explain to parents that regression in this situation is normal and to encourage parents to reinforce appropriate behavior while allowing the regressive behavior to occur.
20. The nurse should ask parents about the toddler's home routines (feeding, bathing, bedtime) and try to adapt hospital routines to which the toddler is accustomed.
21. Because preschoolers lack an understanding of body integrity, they fear mutilation and are afraid of bodily harm from invasive procedures.
22. The nurse can encourage the child to participate in his or her care. This may promote a sense of control. Examples include making menu selections and assisting with treatments when appropriate. The nurse can encourage the child's independence when appropriate.
23. Because peer groups are so important during adolescence, adolescents feel anxiety when separated from their peers. Meeting other hospitalized adolescents can help with this.
24. Regression in toileting or self-feeding skills; temper tantrums; clinging; crying
25. Child's age; level of cognitive development; parent's response to illness or hospitalization; preparation; coping skills
26. Blowing bubbles or singing to promote relaxed breathing; using imagery for the older child; using distraction techniques such as singing, playing games, and listening to music; teaching coping mechanisms and having the child practice them before undergoing a procedure can help a child feel more in control and more relaxed.
27. Increased self-confidence; mastery of self-care skills; learning new information; coping skills
28. They differ in design and intent. Therapeutic play is guided by health team members to help meet the physical and psychological needs of the child.

29. During emotional outlet, or dramatic play, the child acts out or dramatizes real-life stressors.
30. The playroom should have no association with unpleasant experiences, so the child should not receive any treatments (including medications) in the playroom.
31. A reward system can be used in which the child receives a reward when a previously set goal is met. Another example is allowing the child to blow bubbles as a fun way to do deep breathing exercises. See p. 000 in textbook for other examples.
32. Admission should not be a series of questions directed at the child and family but a time of collaboration between nurse and family. The nurse should be aware of the child's and family's needs and should structure the admission process to meet those needs.
33. The immediate physiologic needs of the child; the emotional needs of the child and family.
34. Even parents who feel they are in control of their child before admission find themselves in an unfamiliar environment in the hospital. Parents may be confused as to what they can and cannot do.
35. Jealousy; insecurity; resentment; confusion; anxiety
36. c
37. f
38. d
39. d
40. e
41. b
42. a

Review Questions

1. b
2. c
3. d
4. d
5. a
6. c
7. d
8. c
9. d
10. d

11. b
12. a, c, e
13. d

CHAPTER 12
The Child with a Chronic Condition or Terminal Illness

Student Learning Exercises

1. f
2. d
3. h
4. e
5. a
6. c
7. b
8. g
9. Children with chronic illness are living longer. Advances in medicine have led to children living with illnesses that were previously fatal. Both quality of life and longevity have been enhanced by improvements in diagnostic testing and treatment.
10. Children with special health care needs are those who have, or are at risk for, a chronic physical, developmental, behavioral, or emotional condition and who also require health care and related services of a type and amount beyond that required for children generally.
11. A situational crisis is an unexpected crisis for which the family's usual problem-solving abilities are not adequate.
12. family cohesiveness
13. Reframing a situation to highlight positive rather than negative aspects; successful coping; maintaining high quality communication patterns; being flexible; maintaining social ties; preserving family boundaries
14. F
15. T
16. not only the child but the entire family
17. Denial; anger and resentment; bargaining; sadness or depression; acceptance
18. F

19. T
20. age at onset of the disorder; growth and development
21. self-esteem and self-reliance; autonomy
22. T
23. F
24. To achieve normalization; to achieve and maintain the highest level of physical, emotional, and psychosocial health and function possible.
25. To remain intact; to achieve and maintain normalization; to maximize function
26. Child's physical condition
27. Communication
28. F
29. T
30. T
31. F
32. c
33. a
34. b
35. d
36. T
37. F
38. T
39. Meeting with hospital pastoral care team or personal spiritual counselor; attending nursing support groups mediated by a pastor, social worker, or counselor; participating in patient care conferences or ethics committee meetings
40. Whether to inform the child of the prognosis
41. T
42. T
43. T
44. F
45. T
46. F
47. F
48. T
49. T
50. F

Review Questions
1. a
2. b
3. a
4. b
5. b
6. c
7. d, e, f
8. a
9. c
10. c, d, f

CHAPTER 13
Principles and Procedures for Nursing Care of Children

Student Learning Exercises
1. c
2. f
3. b
4. d
5. a
6. e
7. Child's age; developmental level; personality; current level of knowledge and understanding; past experiences; coping skills; family situation
8. T
9. T
10. T
11. F
12. F
13. T
14. F
15. Age and development of the child; physical condition; destination; safety
16. T
17. T
18. T
19. F
20. Blood; all body fluids, secretions, excretions except sweat; nonintact skin; mucous membranes
21. transmission-based precautions
22. Put alcohol-based rub on hands; rub all over the surface of the hands and fingers; allow to dry thoroughly.
23. 100° F
24. testing the water temperature on the inside of the wrist or elbow
25. three
26. Inhalation of powder into the lungs can cause respiratory complications.
27. T
28. F
29. F
30. There is a risk of aspiration when an infant drinks from a propped bottle.
31. Allow them to sit at a table; allow them to feed themselves; have their parents bring their own utensils from home; use colorful plates and utensils.
32. Take an axillary temperature if the child is less than

4 to 6 years of age or if the child has had oral surgery or is uncooperative, immunosuppressed, or neurologically impaired.
33. The measurement may be inaccurate if liquids were consumed within 30 minutes of measurement, if the child is crying, or if the child is undergoing oxygen therapy or nebulization treatments.
34. The child is younger than 2 years of age; the child has an irregular heartbeat; the child has a congenital heart defect
35. 1 minute
36. 60 seconds
37. 88/P
38. Removing the child's blankets and clothing; lowering the environmental (room) temperature; giving a tepid sponge bath; using a mechanical cooling blanket
39. acetaminophen; ibuprofen
40. standard
41. nasal washing
42. clean
43. posterior iliac crest
44. Tube placement is verified when the tube is inserted, any time the feeding is interrupted, before each bolus feeding, and every 4 to 8 hours during continuous feedings.
45. Auscultation of air entering stomach; aspiration of enteral fluid; pH measurement of the aspirate
46. F
47. F
48. T
49. F
50. 360–480; 3
51. T
52. T
53. It differs very little except for the size of the equipment and the teaching and support of children and families. An oxygen hood can be used for infants, and toddlers and preschoolers can use a nasal cannula, blow-by or face mask. When a humidified environment with oxygen is needed, a cool mist tent can be used.
54. The child has adequate oxygen saturation.

55. Report it to the physician because the child may require oxygen therapy. (For some children with cardiac or respiratory diseases, a pulse oximetry reading of 89% may be normal.)

56. Assessing the stoma area for signs of infection and skin breakdown; changing tracheostomy ties; cleaning the tracheostomy site and inner cannula; changing the tracheostomy tube; suctioning

57. At least every 8 hours

58. 5 seconds

59. off

60. 2 hours before the time of arrival at the hospital.

61. Auscultate lungs to identify any abnormal breath sounds or areas of diminished or absent sounds. Encourage early ambulation, deep breathing, and coughing. Incentive spirometers can increase respiratory movement. To facilitate air exchange, the nurse can engage the child in games such as blowing cotton, a windmill, or bubbles.

62. Separation from significant others; care by strangers; unfamiliar procedures; pain; fear of mutilation; disruption in routine; lack of privacy; temporary disability

Review Questions

1. b
2. a
3. b
4. b
5. c
6. b
7. a
8. d
9. c
10. d
11. d, a, c, e, f, b
12. b
13. b, c, e

CHAPTER 14
Medication Administration and Safety for Infants and Children

Student Learning Exercises

1. c
2. b
3. d
4. f
5. e
6. a
7. Gastric acidity; gastric emptying; gastrointestinal motility; enzyme activity
8. T
9. F
10. F
11. The renal system is immature at birth. The newborn infant's glomerular filtration rate is about 30% to 50% that of an adult, and the renal tubules function less efficiently. Infants and young children cannot concentrate urine as well as older children or adults. Because of renal immaturity medications may not be excreted.
12. When certain medications are used, a peak and trough serum level is measured to monitor medication concentration.
13. trough
14. Nurses should ask parents about medication allergies; child's ability to take medications (e.g., liquid versus solid), and special techniques they use to give medicines; allow parents to administer certain medications (e.g., oral, otic, ophthalmic) if the child will cooperate; ask parents to report if a medication does not seem to be effective
15. Toddler: Give explanations through play; allow the child to see and handle the equipment first; allow the child to help squirt liquid preparations into the mouth; allow the parent to give the medication if the child prefers; use as little restraint as possible because the child will resist restraint; offer praise when the child takes the medication; rewards, such as stickers, are useful.
Preschooler: Offer a choice about what to drink after taking oral medication (limit to two choices);offer a Band-Aid (preferably, a colorful one) after an injection.
School-age child: Offer a choice of drinks when possible (as with preschooler);the child may need a source of distraction to cooperate with painful procedures such as venipuncture or injection; praise for cooperation and use rewards such as stickers

16. F
17. F
18. F
19. Use the six rights of medication administration; double check medication calculations before administration; double check pharmacy calculations of unit dose medications before administration; have two nurses check the following medications: insulin, narcotics, chemotherapy, digoxin, anticoagulants, K^+ and Ca^{++} salts
20. Absorption of oral medications is affected by the presence or absence of food in the stomach, gastric emptying time, gastrointestinal motility, and stomach acidity. It is also less predictable because of medication loss from spillage, leaking, or spitting out.
21. The nurse can check to see whether the medication is available as a liquid. If not, the medications (except those that are enteric coated or sustained release) can be crushed and mixed with a nonessential food such as applesauce.
22. Because medications can alter the flavor of the food, the child may associate that food with the undesirable flavor and refuse it in the future, even without the medication added. Thus, only foods not essential to the child's diet should be used for mixing with medications.
23. F
24. F
25. T
26. T
27. Place the child on her lap with his or her right arm behind the nurse's back and with the nurse's left hand holding the child's left hand. Support the child's head with the nurse's left arm and secure it between the arm and body. Secure the child's legs between the nurse's legs. (Reverse sides if the nurse is left-handed.)

28. Notify the physician and report what medication was vomited and how much time has elapsed since administration.
29. Verify tube is properly positioned before administering medication. Flush tube with water after medication is administered.
30. Explanations should be tailored to the child's cognitive level. Explain the reason for the injection and describe the sensations that the child can expect to feel. The child may need to be assured that the injection is not a punishment for any misbehavior.
31. Ice can be applied to the injection site for several minutes before the injection to numb the area. Children can be taught how to use guided imagery, deep breathing, or distraction to cope with the discomfort. Topical anesthetics such as EMLA cream are effective in reducing injection pain.
32. b
33. c
34. d
35. a
36. T
37. F
38. T
39. F
40. circulation
41. Fat pads above the iliac crests; fat pads above the hips; fat pads above the lateral upper arms; fat pads above the anterior thighs
42. T
43. F
44. F
45. testing (such as allergy testing or purified protein derivative)
46. The inner aspect of the forearm or the upper back
47. Insert needle bevel up at a 15-degree angle. The needle will barely penetrate the skin and when the medication is injected, it will form a wheal.
48. F
49. T
50. T
51. F
52. T
53. F
54. spacer

55. 10 seconds
56. Consider the rate and type of fluid to be administered; the projected length of time the IV will be needed; availability of veins; and the child's developmental level. The child's dominant hand should be avoided as a site for injection.
57. Use guided imagery—for example, putting on a "magic" glove. Try distraction with music, toys, seek-and-find books.
58. Clean the area well and place a liberal amount of cream in a mound on the site. Cover with a transparent occlusive dressing and leave in place for 1 to 2 hours to anesthetize the area.
59. A volumetric pump should be used when IV fluids are administered to prevent inadvertent fluid overload.
60. An IV site should be assessed at least once per hour.
61. Assess for signs of infiltration (edema, erythema, pain, blanching, and coolness) and phlebitis (streaking on the skin above the vein). Discontinue IV if any of these signs is present.
62. 0 to 10 kg: 100 mL/kg/day; 10 to 20 kg: 1000 mL plus 50 mL/kg/day for each kilogram between 10 and 20 kg; >20 kg: 1500 mL plus 20 mL/kg/day for each kilogram >20 kg
63. 1800 mL; 1300 mL
64. These medications are not diluted and are injected (pushed) directly into the IV catheter through the port closest to the patient.
65. It is important to flush the IV tubing to complete the delivery of the medication from the IV tubing into the patient
66. An intermittent infusion port or Heparin lock should be flushed every 6 to 12 hours (to maintain patency).
67. Central venous access devices are used to administer medications, blood products, IV fluids, and parenteral nutrition over the long term to chronically ill children.
68. An implanted venous access device consists of a catheter

that is connected to a port or reservoir. The catheter tip rests at the junction of the superior vena cava and right atrium. The port is under the skin and is accessed with a noncoring needle placed through the skin into the port.
69. phlebitis, infection, and thrombosis
70. F
71. T
72. T
73. Name of the medication; reason it is to be given; action of the medication; expected side effects and what to do if they should occur; when to notify the health care provider; any dietary restrictions; how to take the medication; how to measure the dosage correctly; how to use droppers or syringes

Review Questions

1. a
2. c
3. a
4. d
5. c
6. b
7. c
8. d
9. a, e, d, f
10. c, a, d, b
11. d

CHAPTER 15
Pain Management for Children

Student Learning Exercises

1. c
2. g
3. e
4. b
5. d
6. f
7. a
8. whatever the experiencing person says it is, existing whenever the person says it does
9. an unpleasant sensational and emotional experience associated with actual or potential damage
10. T
11. F
12. F
13. T
14. T

15. the World Health Organization (WHO)
16. the American Pain Society
17. JCAHO
18. T
19. T
20. F
21. F
22. F
23. behavioral; physiologic
24. more purposeful
25. agitation
26. restlessness
27. punishment
28. They fear bodily harm and have an awareness of death.
29. They may not report pain, believing that the nurse must already be aware of it.
30. It is necessary to use pain assessment tools with children in order to provide an objective measure of the pain experience.
31. 3
32. The Oucher and the FACES Pain Rating Scales
33. Regulated breathing techniques are beneficial because they provide a focus for distraction, and they produce relaxation.
34. Children who are distracted can forget the pain, but the pain still exists.
35. relaxation; focused concentration
36. Biofeedback is a technique that allows a person to notice body states not usually noticed and to bring them under control.
37. Muscle relaxation in older children is beneficial because it causes the child to experience relaxation, decreased anxiety, decreased pain, decreased body tension.
38. Hypnosis is a form of focused or narrowed attention, an altered state of consciousness accompanied by relaxation.
39. transmission of pain signals
40. Oxygen; a bag and mask; Naloxone (Narcan)
41. cardiac arrest
42. F
43. T
44. T
45. T
46. F
47. T
48. T

Review Questions

1. a
2. a, c, d
3. b
4. d
5. a
6. c
7. c
8. d
9. d
10. d
11. a, c, f

CHAPTER 16
The Child with a Fluid and Electrolyte Alteration

Student Learning Exercises

1. a
2. c
3. e
4. g
5. b
6. f
7. d
8. h
9. i
10. k
11. j
12. F
13. T
14. F
15. F
16. T
17. extracellular
18. water, solutes
19. sodium; potassium and magnesium
20. 7.35; 7.45
21. Chemical buffers; respiratory system; the kidneys
22. bicarbonate, proteins
23. increase
24. hydrogen ions; bicarbonate
25. b
26. f
27. a
28. e
29. c
30. d
31. a
32. d
33. c
34. b
35. T
36. F
37. T
38. T
39. F
40. T

41. F
42. Diarrhea is an increase in the frequency, fluidity, and volume of stools.
43. gastroenteritis
44. Food intolerance; medications; malabsorption; colon disease; obstruction; irritable bowel syndrome; stress; infectious diseases elsewhere in the body
45. The high carbohydrate content of these drinks may worsen diarrhea. In addition, they do not replace the electrolytes lost through diarrhea.
46. An infant with diarrhea should continue with breast milk or regular strength formula in order to prevent dehydration, to reduce stool frequency and volume, and to reduce duration of diarrhea.
47. Choose from complex carbohydrates (rice, bread, cereals, noodles, potatoes, and crackers), yogurt, cooked vegetables, and lean meats. Avoid beans, spices, fatty foods, sports drinks, colas, apple juice.
48. Change diaper immediately after each bowel movement, wash skin with mild soap and pat dry, apply "barrier" ointment (e.g., A&D ointment), and avoid using commercial baby wipes.
49. T
50. T
51. F
52. F
53. T

Review Questions

1. d
2. b
3. b
4. d
5. a
6. a
7. b
8. c
9. b
10. a
11. d
12. a, d, e, f
13. c

CHAPTER 17
The Child with an Infectious Disease

Student Learning Exercises

1. c
2. h
3. g
4. a
5. b
6. e
7. f
8. d
9. d
10. e
11. b
12. c
13. a
14. skin; intact mucous membranes
15. f
16. c
17. i
18. h
19. a
20. e
21. b
22. j
23. g
24. d
25. k
26. Give the child a lukewarm bath with colloid preparations (Aveeno) or baking soda (½ cup in tub of water); soothing lotions can be applied to the skin; keep child's fingernails short and clean; if the child continues to scratch, put cotton socks or mittens on the child's hands to prevent breaking of the skin and subsequent secondary infections; dress the child in lightweight clothing that is not irritating; antihistamines or antipruritics may be prescribed.
27. T
28. T
29. T
30. T
31. T
32. F
33. F
34. T
35. F
36. F
37. T
38. Ophthalmia neonatorum can be controlled by prophylactic administration of antimicrobial drops immediately after birth.
39. Children with STIs after the neonatal period should be evaluated for sexual abuse.
40. rhinitis; a maculopapular rash; hepatosplenomegaly
41. Infants are infected during the birthing process.
42. Perinatally through aspirated vaginal secretions or through direct contact; through sexual abuse; by voluntary sexual activity
43. d
44. f
45. b
46. a
47. g
48. c
49. e

Review Questions

1. b
2. b
3. b
4. d
5. c
6. c
7. c
8. d
9. a, b, e
10. b
11. b, c, e

CHAPTER 18
The Child with an Immunologic Alteration

Student Learning Exercises

1. d
2. f
3. j
4. i
5. b
6. k
7. h
8. e
9. a
10. g
11. m
12. c
13. l
14. c
15. f
16. i
17. d
18. g
19. b
20. h
21. e
22. a
23. F
24. F
25. T
26. F
27. Through the placenta; during delivery; through breastfeeding
28. zidovudine (ZDV)
29. Administration of trimethoprim-sulfamethoxazole to infants exposed to HIV from about 4–6 months of age to 12 months old, or when the infant is found to be HIV negative.
30. Tanner staging of sexual maturity
31. They decrease monocytes and macrophage differentiation and lymphokine production leading to T-cell inhibition.
32. The child may have acute adrenal insufficiency.
33. ACTH
34. every other day
35. To minimize risk for gastrointestinal bleeding, give corticosteroids with food or milk; to deal with increased appetite, offer low-calorie, low-salt snacks throughout the day
36. Kawasaki disease; poststreptococcal glomerulonephritis
37. Autoantibodies are antibodies that act against the body's own cells.
38. T
39. F
40. T
41. T
42. T
43. F
44. An allergy is an immune response to an antigen (allergen) that causes a hypersensitivity reaction in various body systems.
45. b
46. a
47. d
48. c
49. The most serious features of anaphylaxis are laryngospasm, edema, cyanosis, shock, vascular collapse, cardiac arrest.
50. An Epi-Pen is a preloaded, automatic delivery system of injectable epinephrine available in 0.3 mg (Epi-Pen) and 0.15 mg (Epi-Pen Jr.) doses.

239

51. RAST tests are more expensive. They also provide more precise information about allergies than do skin tests without the risk of hypersensitivity reactions.

Review Questions

1. b
2. c
3. a
4. d
5. b, e
6. c
7. b
8. a
9. b
10. a
11. a, d, e

CHAPTER 19
The Child with a Gastrointestinal Alteration

Student Learning Exercises

1. f
2. j
3. a
4. l
5. g
6. d
7. h
8. k
9. c
10. m
11. e
12. i
13. b
14. n
15. The primary functions of the upper gastrointestinal system are to ingest food and fluids, begin digestion, and propel food to intestines.
16. The primary functions of the lower gastrointestinal system are to digest and absorb nutrients, detoxify and eliminate waste, and maintain fluid and electrolyte balance.
17. Phagocytosis, bile production, detoxification, glycogen storage and breakdown, and vitamin storage are the primary functions of the liver.
18. For the fetus, nutrients are absorbed and waste is excreted through the placenta.
19. T
20. T
21. F

22. T
23. T
24. Polyhydramnios
25. aspiration
26. coughing; cyanosis; choking with feedings
27. Before surgery, an infant with TEF receives nutrition parenterally.
28. Cover stoma with gauze, change gauze often, clean daily with half-strength hydrogen peroxide, use skin barriers.
29. c
30. e
31. b
32. a
33. d
34. f
35. Small, frequent feedings of predigested formulas such as Pregestimil or Nutramigen will reduce the amount of formula in the stomach, decrease distention, and minimize reflux. More frequent feedings with frequent burping are usually the first line of treatment.
36. H$_2$-receptor antagonists, such as cimetidine and ranitidine; prokinetic agents, such as metoclopramide; mucosal protectants, such as sucralfate; proton pump inhibitors, such as omeprazole
37. Over time, the rectum enlarges because of long-term retention of stool. This can result in failure to control the external sphincter, leading to encopresis.
38. Stress
39. diffuse abdominal pain, alternating constipation and diarrhea, undigested food and mucus in stool, normal growth
40. F
41. F
42. T
43. T
44. F
45. T
46. F
47. T
48. F
49. *Crohn disease* can affect any area of the gastrointestinal tract and all its layers. It has periods of remission and exacerbations. Surgery may be required for complications, but

it is not curative. *Ulcerative colitis* affects only the colon and the mucosa and submucosa. It can be cured by a colectomy. See Table 19–4 in the text.
50. Anti-inflammatory agents; antibacterials; antibiotics; immunosuppressive agents
51. The vomiting that occurs with pyloric stenosis is progressive, projectile, non-bilious.
52. stools with bloody mucus, and sausage-shaped abdominal mass
53. Hydrostatic reduction of an intussusception is performed with a barium or air enema or with an ultrasound-guided water enema.
54. Volvulus
55. The cardinal sign of Hirschsprung disease in a newborn infant is delayed passage or absence of meconium stool.
56. enterocolitis
57. T
58. F
59. F
60. T
61. fecal-oral route, contaminated food and water
62. blood, secretions, sexual contact, breast milk
63. blood and blood products
64. blood
65. fecal-oral route
66. *anicteric phase of acute hepatitis:* anorexia, nausea and vomiting, right upper quadrant pain, fever, malaise, irritability, depression; *icteric phase of acute hepatitis:* jaundice, urticaria, dark urine, light-colored stools; *fulminating hepatitis:* bleeding, encephalopathy, ascites, acute hepatic failure
67. Vaccinations are available for HAV and HBV.
68. T
69. F
70. T
71. F
72. T
73. T
74. T
75. ascites, varices, encephalopathy
76. Liver transplantation

1. d
2. b
3. b
4. d
5. b
6. c
7. d
8. a
9. b
10. a
11. b
12. b
13. a, b, e, f
14. b, c, e
15.

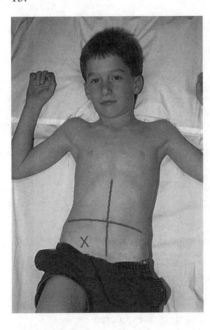

CHAPTER 20
The Child with a Genitourinary Alteration

Student Learning Exercises

1. f
2. d
3. i
4. e
5. j
6. b
7. h
8. g
9. c
10. a
11. abdominal
12. urinary tract infections
13. nephron
14. 10
15. 4.6; 8.0
16. T
17. F

18. T
19. b
20. c
21. d
22. a
23. urine culture
24. suprapubic aspiration
25. vesicoureteral reflux
26. intravenous
27. pyelonephritis
28. Keep foreskin in males clean; cleanse perineal area in girls from front to back; encourage child to urinate at least four times per day; offer fluids throughout day; avoid bubble baths
29. T
30. F
31. T
32. T
33. circumcised
34. epispadias; hypospadias
35. Chordee
36. urethral stents
37. c
38. a
39. e
40. d
41. b
42. The clinical manifestations of acute poststreptococcal glomerulonephritis are hematuria, proteinuria (0 to 2+), edema, renal insufficiency, hypertension
43. They travel through the circulation and get trapped in glomeruli, creating an inflammatory response and damaging the glomeruli. This decreases the glomerular filtration rate, which leads to renal insufficiency.
44. increase
45. Diuresis
46. Proteinuria (3+ to 4+), hypoalbuminemia, edema, anorexia, fatigue, respiratory infection, weight gain, hyperlipidemia
47. Prednisone is used to achieve remission in nephrotic syndrome
48. When urine protein level is 0 to trace for 5 to 7 consecutive days nephrotic syndrome is considered to me in remission.
49. b
50. b
51. a
52. b
53. a

54. c
55. c
56. T
57. T
58. T
59. T
60. waste products; excess body fluids; electrolytes; minerals
61. arteriovenous fistula or graft
62. peritoneal
63. fluid and electrolyte imbalances; acid-base imbalances; osteodystrophy; anemia; poor growth; hypertension; fatigue; decreased appetite; nausea and vomiting; neurologic changes
64. kidney transplantation
65. Rejection
66. the use of immunosuppressive drugs

Review Questions

1. b
2. b, d, e
3. b
4. a
5. d
6. a, b, d, f
7. c
8. a
9. b
10. a
11. c, d, e
12. a
13. b

CHAPTER 21
The Child with a Respiratory Alteration

Student Learning Exercises

1. h
2. m
3. p
4. k
5. b
6. f
7. l
8. o
9. n
10. e
11. q
12. g
13. a
14. j
15. c
16. d
17. i
18. T

19. F
20. T
21. T
22. F
23. T
24. 2 years
25. rhinorrhea; itching eyes, nose, ears, and palate; paroxysmal sneezing; dark circles under eyes; rubbing nose upward with palm of hand
26. A saline solution can be prepared by adding ¼ teaspoon of table salt to 1 cup of warm water.
27. upper respiratory infection
28. acute otitis media with effusion
29. acetaminophen; warm, moist compresses
30. T
31. F
32. T
33. F
34. T
35. F
36. inspiratory stridor with or without retractions
37. a
38. c
39. b
40. d
41. F
42. F
43. T
44. F
45. sudden onset, high fever, sitting in tripod position, nasal flaring and retracting, tachycardia, drooling, dysphagia, dysphonia
46. tongue depressor
47. virus
48. rest; humidification; increased fluid intake
49. 50
50. It can live on the skin for up to an hour and on nonporous surfaces for up to six hours.
51. RSV monoclonal antibody (Synagis)
52. Change position every 2 hours; elevate head of bed; assist older children to cough and deep breathe.
53. 95
54. Nuts; grapes; hard candy; popcorn; hot dogs; raw carrots; large chunks of food
55. aphonia; apnea
56. aspiration, trauma, drug ingestion, shock, massive transfusions
57. Passive smoking

58. Carbon monoxide
59. T
60. F
61. F
62. F
63. b
64. a
65. c
66. time and duration of episode, skin color, heart rate, oxygen saturation, precipitating trigger, any actions taken to stimulate breathing
67. monitor use; cardiopulmonary resuscitation
68. T
69. F
70. T
71. T
72. increased
73. expiration
74. lowers
75. dilate the airway or relieve bronchospasm
76. status asthmaticus
77. Swimming
78. decrease inflammation
79. peak flow meters
80. exposure to triggers
81. T
82. T
83. F
84. T
85. F
86. T
87. F
88. T
89. T
90. T
91. F
92. T
93. a
94. c
95. b
96. T
97. T
98. F
99. F

Review Questions

1. b
2. a
3. b
4. b
5. c
6. c
7. b
8. c
9. a, c
10. b

11. c
12. a
13. d, a, e, c, b, f
14. b, c, d, f
15. a, b, d, e
16. d

CHAPTER 22
The Child with a Cardiovascular Alteration

Student Learning Exercises

1. l
2. g
3. d
4. j
5. c
6. i
7. h
8. k
9. f
10. b
11. a
12. e
13. T
14. T
15. T
16. T
17. F
18. F
19. F
20. T
21. T
22. T
23. placenta
24. foramen ovale
25. ductus arteriosus
26. decreases; increases
27. T
28. F
29. T
30. T
31. T
32. F
33. T
34. F
35. T
36. T
37. F
38. F
39. T
40. T
41. T
42. resting tachycardia and difficulty feeding
43. e
44. b
45. a
46. d
47. c

48. weighing daily
49. the apical heart rate; the dose with another nurse; for signs of digoxin toxicity
50. T
51. T
52. F
53. 85
54. The body attempts to improve tissue oxygenation by increasing the oxygen-carrying capacity of the blood through the production of additional red blood cells.
55. calm the child. Place the child in a knee-chest position; administer oxygen. Morphine may be given to depress the respiratory center and lower the respiratory rate. Vasoconstrictors may be given to increase systemic vascular resistance to decrease right-to-left shunting by forcing blood into the lungs.
56. Indomethacin
57. coarctation of the aorta
58. Ventricular septal defect; atrial septal defect
59. atrioventricular septal defect
60. pulmonary stenosis
61. aortic stenosis
62. f
63. e
64. c
65. a
66. d
67. b
68. g
69. T
70. T
71. F
72. T
73. T
74. F
75. T
76. F
77. T
78. T
79. T
80. F
81. T
82. F
83. T
84. Hypertrophic cardiomyopathy is a major cause of sudden cardiac death.
85. Dilated cardiomyopathy results from an infection or exposure to a toxin.
86. beta; calcium channel blockers

87. Supraventricular tachycardia
88. Hypoxia
89. asystole
90. epinephrine
91. having parents or grandparents who were diagnosed with coronary atherosclerosis before age 55 years; having at least one parent with a total cholesterol level greater than or equal to 240 mg/dL; excessive smoking; decreased exercise; excessive fat intake
92. 170–199; 200

Review Questions

1. a
2. b
3. b, c, d
4. c
5. d
6. a, b, c
7. c
8. d
9. b
10. d
11. a
12. a
13. a, b, e, f
14. d
15. a, b, c

CHAPTER 23
The Child with a Hematologic Alteration

Student Learning Exercises

1. i
2. k
3. f
4. a
5. j
6. h
7. d
8. e
9. c
10. g
11. b
12. a. to transport oxygen to the tissues; b. to destroy foreign cells; c. to prevent blood loss
13. a. decrease in the number of red blood cells or their hemoglobin content; b. increase in number of red blood cells; c. decrease in production of white blood cells; d. source of platelets
14. Cow's milk, which is not iron fortified, replaces formula, which contains additional iron. It may also irritate the immature

bowel, which can lead to gastrointestinal blood loss.
15. They have compromised tissue oxygenation resulting from decreased hemoglobin.
16. Adolescent growth spurt; poor dietary intake; menstruation in females
17. Cow's milk, formula, and cereal can interfere with iron absorption.
18. Low oxygen concentrations; acidosis; dehydration
19. Vaso-occlusion can lead to pain, tissue ischemia, infarcts, organ damage.
20. g
21. f
22. d
23. a
24. e
25. c
26. b
27. autosomal recessive
28. hemosiderosis
29. iron
30. deferoxamine (Desferal)
31. Her father has hemophilia; her mother is a carrier.
32. factor VIII; factor IX
33. Bleeding into the joints can lead to swelling, pain, and stiffness
34. X
35. F
36. T
37. F
38. T
39. T
40. T
41. T
42. F
43. T
44. T
45. T
46. F
47. granulocytes, erythrocytes, megakaryocytes
48. petechiae, ecchymosis, pallor, epistaxis, fatigue, tachycardia, anorexia, and infection
49. colony-stimulating factor
50. A; B
51. negative; positive
52. delivery, miscarriages, and abortions
53. T
54. F
55. F
56. T
57. F

243

1. c
2. b
3. c
4. c
5. c
6. d
7. d
8. d
9. b
10. b
11. b
12. a, c, e

CHAPTER 24
The Child with Cancer

Student Learning Exercises

1. f
2. a
3. h
4. g
5. j
6. c
7. i
8. d
9. b
10. e
11. neoplasm
12. invasion; metastasis
13. Tumor staging describes the extent of the disease locally, regionally, and systemically; it guides therapy for most solid tumors.
14. T
15. F
16. F
17. The signs and symptoms of childhood cancer can depend on type of tumor, extent of disease, child's age
18. chemotherapy; surgery; radiation therapy
19. drugs
20. hematopoietic; gastrointestinal; integumentary
21. The time of greatest bone marrow suppression, generally occurring 7 to 10 days after chemotherapy administration, depending on the specific agent used
22. Neutropenia
23. R
24. B
25. C
26. B
27. C

28. B
29. 5-HT$_3$ serotonin antagonists are drugs that have been found to be effective in treating nausea and vomiting.
30. The purpose of a biopsy is to obtain a small piece of the tumor for microscopic examination for the purpose of confirming tumor type and guiding therapy decisions
31. Provides easy access to venous system. Child does not have to undergo frequent, painful venipunctures.
32. dose; treatment site
33. 7 to 10
34. Erythema within the area being radiated
35. A transplant of a patient's own harvested stem cells.
36. First-remission Philadelphia chromosome-positive acute lymphocytic leukemia, acute myelocytic leukemia, and stage IV neuroblastoma.
37. Preparation for a transplant involving a regimen of chemotherapy, with or without radiation is conditioning.
38. graft-versus-host disease
39. Naturally occurring substances found in small quantities in the body that influence immune system functions are biologic response modifiers.
40. immature white blood cells
41. fever; pallor; excessive bruising; bone or joint pain (usually leg pain); lymphadenopathy; malaise; hepatosplenomegaly; abnormal white blood cell count (either lower or higher than normal for age); mild to profound anemia and thrombocytopenia
42. bone marrow aspiration and biopsy
43. combination chemotherapy
44. Remission is defined as the reduction of immature blast cells in the bone marrow to less than 5%.
45. To decrease serum uric acid levels and alkalinize the urine.
46. Risk for Infection related to immunosuppressed state; Risk for Injury related to thrombocytopenia; Imbalanced

Nutrition: Less than Body Requirements related to nausea and vomiting, mucositis, or taste changes; Deficient Knowledge related to unfamiliarity with the disease process and treatment plan; Disturbed Body Image related to hair loss; Ineffective Individual/Family Coping related to chronic illness; Acute and Chronic Pain related to the disease process and procedures
47. A rectal thermometer can damage delicate rectal tissues, resulting in infection.
48. 500 cells/mm^3
49. Use a soft-bristled toothbrush, perform oral hygiene four times a day, and at the first sign of mouth ulcers, notify physician to begin using an antifungal medication. Do not use alcohol-containing mouthwashes.
50. Giving a live-virus vaccine to an immunosuppressed child could produce infection.
51. Give the child varicella-zoster immune globulin within 96 hours of exposure.
52. Limit activities to prevent injury, particularly to the head; no contact sports; use a soft-bristled toothbrush or gauze swab to clean teeth; give stool softeners but no suppositories; check urine and stools for blood; teach child how to control nosebleeds and to blow the nose gently; adolescent girls should monitor their menstrual flow.
53. Cool, clear liquids and soft, bland foods at room temperature should be offered to a nauseated child.
54. F
55. F
56. T
57. F
58. T
59. tumor location; age and development of the child
60. Headaches and morning vomiting related to getting out of bed are the two hallmark symptoms of brain tumors in children.
61. magnetic resonance imaging

62. Surgery and chemotherapy are used to treat brain tumors in children.
63. This position increases intracranial pressure and the risk of bleeding.
64. increased intracranial pressure
65. F
66. F
67. T
68. F
69. T
70. T
71. F
72. T
73. T

Review Questions

1. a
2. d
3. c
4. b
5. c
6. a
7. c
8. b
9. c
10. b
11. a
12. a
13. a
14. b
15. a
16. b, d, f
17. c
18. a, c, f

CHAPTER 25
The Child with Major Alterations in Tissue Integrity

Student Learning Exercises

1. k
2. d
3. i
4. h
5. e
6. b
7. j
8. f
9. a
10. c
11. g
12. Protects deeper tissues from injury, drying, and foreign matter invasion; regulates temperature; aids in excretion of wastes; produces vitamin D; initiates the sensations of touch, pain, heat, and cold
13. T
14. T
15. F
16. F
17. impetigo
18. *Staphylococcus aureus*
19. Bullous impetigo presents as small vesicles that can progress to bullae. The lesions are initially filled with serous fluid and later become pustular. The bullae rupture, leaving a shiny, lacquered-appearing lesion surrounded by a scaly rim. Crusted impetigo appears initially as a vesicle or pustule, which ruptures to become an erosion with an overlay of honey-colored crust. When crusts are removed, the erosion bleeds easily.
20. Failure to respond to treatment indicates the infection is caused by community-acquired methicillin-resistant *S. aureus.*
21. Impetigo is treated with topical and oral antibiotics. Wash lesions three times a day with a warm, soapy washcloth. Then apply topical antibiotics. Severe cases or cases of impetigo around the mouth are treated with oral antibiotics.
22. Acute glomerulonephritis is a complication of impetigo caused by beta-hemolytic streptococci.
23. The child should sleep alone and be bathed alone with antibacterial soap. The caregiver should wear gloves when caring for the child. Complete the full course of antibiotics.
24. Cellulitis is a bacterial infection of the subcutaneous tissues and dermis.
25. The lower extremities and buccal and periorbital regions are the body parts most commonly affected by cellulitis.
26. Affected areas will appear red, hot, swollen, and painful; lymphangitis will occur with red streaking of the surrounding area; edema and purple discoloration of eyelids appear with decreased eye movement if the periorbital area is affected; and lymph node enlargement, fever, malaise, and headache occur.
27. Cellulitis is treated by administering an initial intramuscular or intravenous dose of an antibiotic, then complete a 10-day course of antibiotics and warm compresses. Hospitalization and intravenous antibiotics are required if cellulitis affects a joint or the face. Incision and drainage of the affected area may be necessary.
28. Have the child rest in bed with the affected leg elevated; warm moist soaks should be applied every four hours; administer antibiotics as ordered; acetaminophen can be given for fever or pain; assess for signs of sepsis or spread of infection; practice frequent handwashing
29. *Candida albicans* is the organism responsible for causing thrush.
30. Thrush manifests as white, curd-like plaques on the tongue, gums, or buccal membranes that are difficult to remove.
31. Does she have vaginal itching or discharge? Does she have any tenderness or redness of the nipples? Ask about her methods of cleaning bottles, nipples, and pacifiers and about the infant's prior feeding patterns.
32. Nystatin oral suspension is medication used to treat oral candidiasis.
33. Swab 1 mL of oral nystatin suspension onto the infant's gums and tongue every 6 hours until 3 to 4 days after symptoms have disappeared. The parent can rub the suspension onto mucous membranes with a gloved hand.
34. a: scalp; b: trunk, face, and extremities; c: feet
35. a: griseofulvin orally for 6 weeks; b: antifungal preparations such as clotrimazole (Lotrimin) or miconazole (Monistat) topically three times a day to affected area until lesions are gone for 1 week; c: topical antifungal

245

preparation applied twice daily to lesions and at least 1 inch beyond lesion borders; d: topical antifungal agent such as clotrimazole (Lotrimin), miconazole (Monistat), or oxiconazole (Oxistat) applied twice daily until lesions have been cleared for 1 week.

36. T
37. F
38. F
39. HSV-1 infection of the fingers that is transmitted during oral or tracheal care of a child with herpes infection.
40. Oral or topical acyclovir (Zovirax) can lessen the severity of HSV-1.
41. The mother can try to feed the child frozen ice pops, noncitrus juices, milk, or flat soda. Small, frequent meals of soft, bland foods may be tolerated. Reassure parent that a few days without solid food is not harmful as long as fluid intake is adequate.
42. F
43. F
44. Nits are visible silvery, gray-white specks resembling dandruff that are firmly attached to the hair shafts near the scalp. Nits resemble dandruff but are more difficult to remove from the hair. They are commonly found ¼- to ½-inch from the scalp surface behind the ears and at the nape of the neck.
45. After the hair is treated with a pediculocide, all nits must be removed from the hair; the child should be rechecked in 7 to 10 days for infestation; parents should be advised to wash clothing, bedding, and linens in hot water and to dry at a hot dryer setting; items that cannot be washed can be dry cleaned or sealed in plastic bags for two to three weeks; thorough home cleaning is necessary to remove any hairs that might carry live nits; combs and brushes should be boiled or soaked in antilice shampoo or hot water (>140° F) for at least 10 minutes

46. Scabies is transmitted by close personal contact with infected individuals.
47. Clinical manifestations of scabies are: intense itching, especially at night; papules, vesicles, and nodules on the wrists, finger webs, elbows, umbilicus, axillae, groin, and buttocks; presence of burrows (fine, grayish, threadlike lines) that are difficult to see because of inflammation and excoriation from scratching.
48. A topical application is applied to the body and head, avoiding the eyes and mouth. Lotion is kept on the body for the recommended period of time (usually 8 to 14 hours) and then the child is bathed.
49. asthma; allergic rhinitis
50. High levels of histamine trigger an inflammatory response resulting in erythema, edema, and intense pruritus. Scratching increases itching, leading to an "itch-scratch itch" cycle.
51. Rash on the flexor surfaces of the wrists, ankles, knees and elbows, neck creases, eyelids, and dorsum of hands and feet. Chronic lichenification results from persistent scratching. Areas may be weeping and possibly infected.
52. Apply moisturizing cream several times a day and immediately after bathing to hydrate the skin; avoid trigger factors such as overheating, soaps, wool clothing, or any skin irritant; keep child's fingernails short; cotton gloves or mittens might be needed at night
53. cradle cap
54. Nonpruritic oily yellow scales on the scalp, forehead, eyebrows, and behind the ears; confluent erythema in the diaper area and intertriginous areas and around the umbilicus
55. Remove scales daily by shampooing with a mild baby shampoo or an over-the-counter antiseborrheic shampoo containing sulfur and salicylic acid, selenium, or tar; massage the scalp with warm mineral oil

before shampooing to loosen the scales; use a fine-toothed comb or clean soft-bristled toothbrush to loosen the scales.
56. Contact dermatitis is a skin inflammation that results from direct skin-to-irritant contact.
57. Cool compresses; antipruritic lotions; Aveeno baths; topical steroid creams; oral antihistamines
58. Rinse the child's skin with cool water immediately and wash clothing in hot, soapy water.
59. T
60. T
61. T
62. Sebaceous hair follicles on the face, neck, back, shoulders, and upper chest
63. When the sebaceous or sweat glands become blocked, a blackhead or a pimple is formed. If these rupture under the skin, inflammation occurs.
64. a. Avoid exposure to sunlight; b. If sexually active, use contraception because of the drug's teratogenic effect on the fetus.
65. Wash the face twice a day with an antibacterial soap and shampoo hair daily. Avoid vigorous scrubbing and picking or squeezing pimples. Use only water-based cosmetics. Get adequate rest and exercise, and eat a balanced diet.
66. Wear identification describing the allergy and stating the treatment. Keep an emergency kit containing antihistamine, epinephrine, and a syringe available.
67. If the stinger is in the skin, it can be removed by carefully scraping it out horizontally. Do not squeeze the area, because more venom will be released. Wash with soap and water. A meat tenderizer paste applied to the area may be soothing, ice and analgesics for discomfort and antihistamines for itching.
68. Insect repellants containing DEET shouldn't be used on children because of the risk for toxic encephalopathy.
69. Cover affected areas immediately with warm hands and clothing. Do not

massage the area. Rewarm by immersion in a warm bath (90°–106° F) until all parts are thawed and the skin appears flushed.

70. Child should wear warm, layered clothing, hat, gloves, and two pairs of socks (one wool, one cotton). Teach children to warm their hands and feet when they begin to sting. Do not allow young children to play in extremely cold temperatures.

71. Remove with tweezers as close to the skin as possible, taking care to remove the head. If mouth parts remain, remove with sterile needle. Wash area with soap and water.

72. d
73. a
74. b
75. c
76. b
77. a
78. b
79. c
80. c
81. a
82. b
83. c

84. Avoid sun exposure, especially between 10 AM and 3 PM during the summer. Apply ultraviolet A and ultraviolet B protective sunscreens with SPF >15 to the child's skin. Apply frequently. Use a waterproof sunscreen if children are in and out of water. Wear a hat and a shirt. Sunscreen is contraindicated for infants under age 6 months. Infants should be kept in the shade away from reflecting sun rays.

85. Silver nitrate solution; mafenide acetate cream; silver sulfadiazine cream

86. Burn shock is a hypovolemic condition that develops after burn injury affecting more than 15% to 20% of total body surface area.

87. Cardiac arrest or arrhythmia; tissue damage; myoglobinuria; metabolic acidosis

88. scalding liquids.

Review Questions

1. b
2. a
3. c
4. c
5. d
6. b
7. d
8. b
9. b
10. c
11. d
12. a
13. b
14. a
15. c
16. a, b, d
17. a

CHAPTER 26
The Child with a Musculoskeletal Alteration

Student Learning Exercises

1. c
2. e
3. i
4. h
5. a
6. g
7. d
8. b
9. f
10. T
11. F
12. T
13. T
14. T
15. F
16. 16–18
17. A large amount of force is necessary to fracture the bone. Abuse or an underlying pathologic condition is often the cause.
18. immobilize
19. continuous
20. 30 pounds; 2–3 years
21. skeletal
22. Osteomyelitis
23. Pain; paresthesia; pallor; pulselessness; paralysis
24. check that correct weight is applied; weights are hanging freely and not touching the floor or bed; ropes are appropriately on the pulleys; assess neurovascular status regularly
25. T

26. T
27. T
28. F
29. T
30. T
31. F
32. a. femoral head that can be displaced with manipulation, asymmetric gluteal skin folds; limited range of motion with asymmetric abduction of hip; and shorter-appearing femur on affected side; b. gait variation with lurching toward affected side; limited abduction on affected side(s)
33. The Pavlik harness maintains the hip in the following positions: abduction, flexion, external rotation
34. avascular necrosis
35. Harness straps secure enough to keep hips flexed; harness is worn 23 hours and is removed according to physician instructions; place a long tee shirt or onesie under the harness to protect skin; diaper should go under harness; inspect skin for irritation; reposition frequently
36. T
37. T
38. F
39. F
40. above
41. Persistent hip pain, limp, thigh or knee soreness or stiffness
42. child abuse
43. bone growth
44. airway, breathing, and circulation
45. emboli
46. Compartment syndrome is a serious complication occurring when swelling causes pressure to rise within the closed space of an extremity. The increased pressure compromises circulation to muscles and nerves, causing paralysis and necrosis.
47. retention
48. internal fixation
49. d
50. c
51. b
52. a
53. swelling
54. neurovascular impairment; diminished range of motion

247

55. Repetitive stress from sports; overuse of immature muscles and tendons; imbalance in strength of quadriceps muscle
56. insidious onset of knee pain; swelling of the tibial tubercle; difficulty with weight bearing
57. An inherited disorder characterized by connective tissue and bone defects.
58. Osteoporosis; bone fragility and fractures; blue sclerae; discolored teeth; deafness by age 20–30 years
59. T
60. T
61. F
62. T
63. Monitor intravenous site for complications; have thorough knowledge of the antibiotic being given; calculation of safe dosage; determine whether serum levels are therapeutic; review laboratory data on liver and kidney function, complete blood cell count, and erythrocyte sedimentation rate
64. Juvenile arthritis is an autoimmune inflammatory disease that affects the body's connective tissue.
65. Inflammation of the eye structure in the uveal tract
66. Slow-acting antirheumatic drugs are used when children with severe juvenile arthritis do not respond well to nonsteroidal anti-inflammatory drugs.
67. chronic pain related to the inflammatory process
68. progressively degenerative; inherited
69. Duchenne
70. Cardiopulmonary complications are the most common cause of death resulting from muscular dystrophy.
71. T
72. T
73. T
74. T

Review Questions
1. c
2. c
3. a
4. b

5. a
6. c
7. a
8. b
9. c
10. a
11. a
12. d
13. d
14. c
15. a
16. a, b, c
17. d
18. c, a, b, d **or** a, b, d, c

CHAPTER 27
The Child with an Endocrine or Metabolic Alteration

Student Learning Exercises
1. b
2. e
3. a
4. f
5. h
6. g
7. c
8. d
9. b
10. a
11. a
12. a
13. b
14. a
15. a
16. Alterations in endocrine functioning is diagnosed by laboratory testing.
17. height; weight
18. 40 mg/dL
19. premature; small for gestational age
20. Jitteriness; poor feeding; lethargy; seizures; hypotonia; high-pitched cry; bradycardia; cyanosis; temperature instability; respiratory alterations, including apnea
21. Feed formula, breast milk, or D5W. Frequent glucose checks are done to monitor response.
22. If a neonate is at increased risk for hypoglycemia, the nurse should assess gestational age; infant's weight, length, and head circumference plotted on growth curve; blood glucose level by 2 hours of age.

23. A complication that can occur when a neonate is receiving intravenous glucose is that infiltration of the IV can cause severe extravasation.
24. 7.0 mg/dL
25. Maternal diabetes causes immature parathyroid function in the neonate.
26. Autosomal recessive
27. Central nervous system
28. Testing should be done after the infant is 48 hours old.
29. Phenylketonuria can be treated with a special diet that restricts phenylalanine intake (low-phenylalanine diet).
30. F
31. T
32. F
33. glucocorticoids; androgens
34. Ambiguous genitalia in an infant would raise suspicion of congenital adrenal hyperplasia.
35. glucocorticoid therapy
36. F
37. T
38. T
39. T
40. F
41. a
42. b
43. b
44. a
45. a
46. a
47. antithyroid therapy with propylthiouracil or methimazole
48. Neutropenia; hepatotoxicity; hypothyroidism
49. Ineffective Therapeutic Regimen Management related to nonadherence to medication; Diarrhea related to increased basal metabolic rate; Risk for Activity Intolerance related to loss of muscle mass from increased basal metabolic rate; Disturbed Sleep Pattern related to increased basal metabolic rate; Ineffective Thermoregulation related to increased basal metabolic rate
50. vasopressin or antidiuretic hormone
51. Increased urination (polyuria); excessive thirst (polydipsia)

52. The normal response to a water deprivation test is decreased urine output with high specific gravity and no change in serum sodium. In diabetes insipidus, when fluid is restricted, the child continues to produce large amounts of dilute urine (as evidenced by low urine specific gravity) and the serum sodium level may increase.
53. Synthetic vasopressin
54. The medication is administered intranasally or by subcutaneous injection.
55. The kidneys reabsorb too much free water.
56. a. decreased; b. increased; c. decreased; d. retained
57. seizures
58. Premature appearance of secondary sexual characteristics, accelerated growth rate, and advanced bone maturation
59. Rapid bone growth, which causes early fusion and ultimately results in short adult stature.
60. administration of a gonadotropin-releasing hormone agonist or blocker
61. It inhibits binding of gonadotropin-releasing hormone to the pituitary gland, causing a decrease in hormone production. This slows or stops sexual development from progressing.
62. F
63. F
64. T
65. T
66. glucose
67. glycogen
68. to regulate blood glucose by controlling the rate of glucose uptake by cells
69. An autoimmune process that results in destruction of the insulin-secreting cells of the pancreas
70. When glucose is unable to move into the intercellular space, hyperglycemia occurs.
71. Glucose spills into the urine by osmotic diuresis, causing increased urination.
72. Excess fluid is lost through polyuria, causing thirst.

73. Cellular starvation from lack of glucose causes hunger.
74. Cellular starvation from lack of glucose causes weight loss.
75. a
76. c
77. c
78. d
79. b
80. c
81. 120 mg/dL; 200 mg/dL
82. Insulin is a protein and would be digested if taken orally.
83. Measure blood glucose at least four times per day; be able to count carbohydrates; calculate insulin coverage; supportive home environment
84. F
85. F
86. T
87. T
88. T
89. F
90. F
91. T
92. Toddler/preschooler: Chooses and cleans finger for puncture, helps by holding still for injection, identifies words or phrase to describe feeling of hypoglycemia. School-age child: Performs finger puncture and blood glucose test, chooses injection site according to rotation schedule, pushes plunger on syringe after parent inserts needle, performs ketone test. Early adolescent: Records blood glucose values in diary, draws up insulin with supervision, and gives injection. Middle/late adolescent: Prepares and gives insulin injection, looks for patterns in blood glucose values, recognizes when to test for ketones, initiates treatment for ketones.
93. Hypoglycemia could result from a missed or delayed meal, too much insulin, or an unusual amount of exercise without increasing carbohydrate intake.
94. Rub a small amount of glucose gel on the inner cheek and gums, or inject glucagon subcutaneously or intramuscularly. Inject 1 mg for

the child weighing more than 50 pounds or 20 to 30 units/kg for the child weighing less than 50 pounds. Position the unconscious child on their side. Once child is conscious, replace lost glycogen stores with a large snack.
95. a. elevated; b. large; c. low; d. low, normal, or elevated
96. It is necessary to replace fluids lost from diuresis as a result of hyperglycemia. Fluids are essential in flushing ketones.
97. This deep and rapid breathing is a mechanism for removing excess acetone.
98. Regular insulin administered intravenously.
99. Always give the insulin injection, even if the child does not have an appetite; test blood glucose at least every 4 hours; test for urinary ketones with each voiding; offer the child calorie-free liquids; follow the child's usual meal plan; encourage rest; notify physician of nausea and vomiting, fruity odor to the breath, deep, rapid respirations, decreasing level of consciousness, moderate to high urinary ketones, persistent hyperglycemia.
100. T
101. F
102. F

Review Questions
1. c
2. c
3. d
4. b
5. b
6. d
7. a
8. d
9. b
10. c
11. b
12. c
13. b
14. a
15. a
16. b
17. a, b, e, f
18. b
19. c, d, e

249

Student Learning Exercises

1. c
2. d
3. g
4. e
5. a
6. f
7. b
8. a. fourth week; b. 15–20 weeks; c. 30 weeks and continuing to 1 year of age; d. 16 weeks
9. Cerebrum; cerebellum; brainstem
10. The cerebrospinal fluid acts as a watery cushion surrounding the brain to reduce the force of trauma on the brain.
11. b
12. d
13. e
14. f
15. a
16. c
17. a. identify abnormal tissue and structures, such as tumor, bleeding, or hydrocephalus
    b. identify abnormal electrical brain discharges, as in seizures
    c. measure cerebrospinal fluid pressure, identify infection, and administer medication
    d. visualize morphologic features and structures of the brain at a detailed level
18. Ineffective Cerebral Tissue Perfusion; Imbalanced Nutrition: Less than Body Requirements; Risk for Impaired Skin Integrity; Parental Anxiety; Deficient Knowledge
19. Venous outflow drainage of the brain is facilitated by gravity.
20. A prone position, a flexed neck, and hip flexion should be avoided because they raise intracranial pressure.
21. Neurologic impairment can result in difficulty swallowing or chewing and increases the risk of aspiration. Nausea and vomiting are symptoms of several neurologic impairments.

22. a. bulging fontanel, high-pitched cry, poor feeding, vomiting, irritability, restlessness, distended scalp veins, eyes deviated downward, increased head circumference, separation of cranial sutures
    b. headache, diplopia, mood swings, slurred speech, nausea and vomiting (especially in the morning), altered level of consciousness, papilledema (after 48 hours)
23. Decorticate; decerebrate
24. Eye opening; verbal response; motor response
25. b
26. d
27. c
28. f
29. a
30. e
31. T
32. F
33. F
34. F
35. failure of the neural tube to close, resulting in incomplete closure of vertebrae
36. a. sac-like protrusion filled with spinal fluid and meninges
    b. sac filled with spinal fluid, meninges, nerve roots, and spinal cord
37. T
38. T
39. F
40. T
41. T
42. T
43. placement of a ventriculoperitoneal shunt
44. a
45. c
46. b
47. b
48. a
49. c
50. d
51. b
52. c
53. a
54. F
55. T
56. T
57. Equipment includes suction, oxygen, Ambu Bag and mask, and padding of side rails. Pillows should not be used to pad the side rails because they may cause suffocation.

58. Motor vehicle collisions; falls; sports injuries; child abuse; neglect
59. Evaluation of airway, breathing, and circulation (ABCs) are included in the assessment of a child with a head injury.
60. Notify the physician if bleeding does not stop after 10 minutes of holding pressure, if the wound requires sutures, if the child is <1 year of age, if the child has a seizure after head injury, if the child is unconscious or confused, or if the child has any of the following: severe headache, vomiting, slurred speech, blurred vision, difficulty walking or crawling, blood or watery drainage from nose or ear, unequal pupils or crossed eyes.
61. An after-effect of a head injury—the child may upset easily, be irritable if tired or stressed.
62. c
63. a
64. e
65. b
66. d
67. T
68. F
69. T
70. T
71. T
72. a
73. d
74. b
75. c
76. A seizure occurs when there is an excessive disorderly discharge of neuronal activity in the brain. Epilepsy refers to recurrent seizure activity that does not occur in association with an acute illness.
77. Excessive neuronal discharges activate motor or sensory organs. The extent of the seizure depends on the location and extent of abnormal neuronal discharges.
78. height, rapidity
79. Precipitating events; behavior before and immediately after the seizure; detailed description of how the seizure progressed; and the duration of the seizure.

80. Pad side rails; keep the bed in a low position; suction and airway at child's bedside; remove sharp objects or furniture from the area; do not put anything in to the child's mouth; place child on his or her side; do not restrain the child; place on a soft surface if not in bed; loosen clothing around the neck.

81. Gums may become swollen and tender; brush and floss teeth after every meal with a soft toothbrush; have a dental examination every 3 to 6 months; and have blood levels monitored regularly.

82. Prolonged seizure activity that may be a single seizure lasting 10 minutes or recurrent seizures lasting more than 30 minutes with no return to consciousness between seizures.

83. Lumbar puncture

84. Pain with extension of leg and knee

85. Flexion of head causes flexion of hips and knees.

86. Antibiotic therapy; child is placed in a private room on droplet transmission precautions until he or she receives 24 hours of antibiotic therapy

87. T

88. T

89. F

90. Infiltration of lymphocytes in peripheral nerves, causing inflammation.

91. respiratory, neurologic

92. Ineffective Breathing Pattern; Decreased Cardiac Output; Risk for Impaired Skin Integrity; Impaired Verbal Communication; Impaired Urinary Elimination; Anxiety; Deficient Knowledge; Interrupted Family Processes

93. Stress; food; menstruation; visual stimuli; fatigue; certain medications

94. They differ in etiology and manifestations.

Review Questions

1. a
2. b
3. d, e, f
4. c
5. c
6. d

7. c
8. a
9. a
10. d
11. a
12. a
13. b
14. c
15. d
16. c
17. c
18. c
19. a, c, e, f
20. c
21. b

CHAPTER 29
The Child and Family with Psychosocial Alterations

Student Learning Exercises

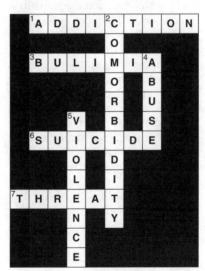

8. F
9. T
10. a. to assess for specific drugs excreted by the kidneys; b. to assess for long-term effects of malnutrition, evidence of specific drugs, and potency of selected medications prescribed for treatment; c. to identify current and previous fractures that may be suggestive of physical abuse; d. indicator of malnutrition when physical neglect is suspected; e. to determine whether sexual abuse has occurred
11. f
12. c

13. b
14. a
15. e
16. d
17. F
18. T
19. T
20. Selective serotonin reuptake inhibitors
21. Using cryptic verbal messages; giving away personal items; changes in expected patterns of behaviors; specific statements about suicide or self-harm; preoccupation with death; frequent risk-taking or self-abusive behaviors; use of drugs or alcohol to cope; overwhelming sense of guilt or shame; obsessional self-doubt; open signs of mental illness; history of physical or sexual abuse; homosexuality; significant change or life event that is internally disruptive
22. Have you ever thought of trying to hurt yourself? How might you do this? Have you ever thought of trying to kill yourself? How might you do this? Have you ever told anyone about wanting to kill yourself? How do you feel right now? Do you have access to firearms? Knives? (For more questions, see Box 29-1.)
23. Communicate with the adolescent in an empathetic and nonjudgmental way to decrease his or her sense of isolation and rejection. Use clear, direct, and supportive tone of voice and demeanor. Be physically and emotionally present, and offer opportunities for him or her to discuss feelings and thoughts. Remove any potentially harmful objects.
24. T
25. F
26. F
27. T
28. Deliberate refusal to maintain adequate body weight; distorted body image; amenorrhea
29. Recurrent episodes of binge eating; a sense of lack of control over eating binges; self-induced vomiting or excessive use of laxatives, diuretics, or emetics to prevent weight gain;

251

excessive exercise to prevent weight gain; a persistent over concern with body image
30. T
31. T
32. T
33. F
34. Attention and concentration; impulse control; overactivity
35. On the basis of reports by the child, parent(s), and teacher(s)
36. to teach the family about the disorder.
37. F
38. T
39. T
40. F
41. F
42. Substances that an adolescent might use initially, such as beer or wine, then progress to cigarettes or hard liquor, move to marijuana and then other illicit drugs.
43. Increase in antisocial behavior; poor school performance; irregular school attendance; aggressive or rebellious behavior; excessive influence by peers; deterioration of relationships with family or former friends; history of lack of parental support and supervision; rapid or extreme changes in mood; loss of interest in hobbies; changes in eating or sleeping patterns as manipulative behaviors increase
44. T
45. F
46. T
47. W: wakefulness, I: irritability, T: tremulousness, temperature variation, tachypnea, H: hyperactivity, high-pitched persistent cry, hyperacusia, hyperreflexia, hypertonus, D: diarrhea, diaphoresis, dehydration, disorganized suck, R: respiratory distress, rub marks, rhinorrhea, A: apnea, autonomic dysfunction, W: weight loss or failure to gain weight, A: alkalosis (respiratory), L: lacrimation
48. Organize care to limit the number of times the infant is disturbed; keep noise level to a minimum; darken the area by placing a light blanket over the top of the incubator; provide comfort measures immediately when the infant becomes irritable.
49. Isolation from community and social groups; intense competition for emotional resources within family; low levels of differentiation among family members; distrust of outsiders and family members; unpredictable and unstable family environment. (For more characteristics, see Box 29-00.)
50. Vigorous shaking while the infant is being held by the extremities or shoulders, causing whiplash-induced intracranial or intraocular bleeding.
51. It is a form of physical abuse in which the caretaker (usually the mother) falsifies or produces illness in the child and then takes the child in for medical care, claiming no knowledge of how the child became ill.
52. Provide an accepting environment; use role modeling as a method of parent teaching; focus on child's positive attributes; encourage parents to participate in child's care; to reinforce positive behavior
53. T
54. F
55. T

Review Questions
1. d
2. a
3. c
4. a
5. b
6. d
7. c
8. b
9. a, b, e
10. d

CHAPTER 30
The Child with a Developmental Disability

Student Learning Exercises
1. c
2. b
3. d
4. a
5. intelligence; adaptive
6. Manifests before 18 years; includes significant sub-average general intellectual functioning; has concurrent deficits in two or more adaptive areas, such as communication, home living, community use, health and safety, leisure, self-care, social skills, self-direction, functional academics, and work
7. Severe and chronic disability that is attributable to mental or physical impairment or to a combination of both; impairment present before age 22 years; impairment likely to continue, resulting in the need for life-long individual services or supports; substantial functional limitations in three or more areas
8. This law required states to provide an education for all disabled children ages 3 to 21 years that is free and appropriate and in the least restrictive environment.
9. Each child with a disability must have a written individualized education program that outlines specialized instruction and services the school system must provide. It is designed by the child's parents and school personnel after an educational assessment.
10. Intense stress felt by families of disabled children; parental isolation; unrealistic expectations for the child's performance resulting from a lack of knowledge about normal growth and development
11. Delayed achievement of developmental milestones
12. Down syndrome; fragile X syndrome
13. T
14. T
15. T
16. F
17. T
18. Risk for Injury related to level of self-care skills and inability to anticipate danger; Deficient Knowledge related

to unfamiliarity with the cause and likely outcomes of the child's cognitive disabilities, available support systems, or information about sexuality, vocational options, leisure skills, and so on; Impaired Social Interaction related to an inability to initiate and maintain social relationships; Compromised or Disabled Family Coping related to excessive emotional and financial strain on family members caring for a cognitively impaired individual, lack of acceptance by society, or an extended grieving process associated with a diagnosis of a child with a chronic disability

19. at home until early adulthood, after which group home placement is an option
20. characteristic features
21. The child's typical coping patterns; daily routines; understanding of language; learning abilities; social and motor skills; environment
22. T
23. F
24. F
25. T
26. T
27. F
28. F
29. Short palpebral fissures, smooth philtrum, and thin upper lip
30. neurologic; developmental
31. F
32. pervasive developmental disorder
33. Disturbance in the rate and appearance of physical, social, and language skills; abnormal responses to body sensations; presence of thinking capacity, but with absent or delayed speech and language; abnormal ways of relating to people, objects, and events
34. A lack of social interaction and awareness.
35. F
36. F
37. F
38. F
39. a
40. c

41. a
42. c
43. b
44. a, d
45. b
46. d
47. A maladaptive parent-infant relationship in which the parent displays impaired skills in reading or responding to the infant's cues.
48. Weight below the 5th percentile, a sudden or rapid deceleration on the growth curve, delay in reaching developmental milestones, and decreased muscle mass. Additional signs include muscle hypotonia, abdominal distention, generalized weakness, and cachexia.
49. Avoidance of eye contact and physical touch, intense watchfulness, sleep disturbances, lack of age-appropriate stranger anxiety or preference for own parents, and disturbed affect.
50. Feed on demand and increase amount as tolerated. For the infant eating solid foods, offer high-protein snacks between meals, offer small portions of a wide variety of foods, and decrease distractions during mealtime. Plan naps so that infant is rested for meals. Intervene when the infant is fretful or crying so that caloric expenditure does not exceed intake.
51. T
52. T

Review Questions

1. d
2. c
3. d
4. a
5. c
6. b
7. b
8. a
9. c
10. c
11. c
12. d
13. b, d, e
14. a

CHAPTER 31
The Child with a Sensory Alteration

Student Learning Exercises

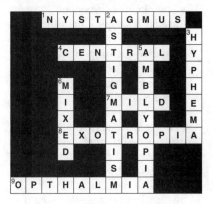

10. f
11. g
12. a
13. c
14. d
15. h
16. b
17. e
18. i
19. 22–50
20. 4–6
21. 6 months
22. 4 to 6
23. hearing
24. d
25. b
26. h
27. f
28. i
29. e
30. a
31. c
32. g
33. prevention; early detection
34. safety
35. Excessive tearing, crusting, or matter on the eyelids on awakening
36. After washing hands thoroughly, place index finger over the lacrimal duct and gently massage in an upward motion.
37. Correction to 20/200 or less in the better eye or a visual field of 20 degrees or less
38. Squinting, frowning, moving objects so they can be seen more easily

253

39. 3 years
40. Permanent loss of vision
41. It strengthens the weak eye while the good eye is patched.
42. Complaints of frequent headaches, squinting, tilting head to see
43. Excessive tearing, light sensitivity, muscle spasm causing involuntary closing of the eyelid
44. surgery
45. Pain, nausea and vomiting, and increased inflammation
46. Elevate the head of the bed slightly and avoid any position in which the affected eye is dependent because this would cause edema and pressure on the eye.
47. Itching; burning; light sensitivity; scratchy eyelids; redness; edema; discharge
48. Chemical irritation from eye prophylaxis
49. Practice good handwashing habits, do not share the child's linens or eye medication with other family members, and do not allow child to return to school or day care until he or she has received eye drops for 24 hours.
50. Administer prescribed medications; assess intravenous site; monitor for signs that infection is spreading with a neurological assessment; pain assessment; hot packs

four times a day; administer analgesics as needed
51. wearing protective eyewear, such as goggles and face masks
52. Reduces the risk of rebleeding between 3 and 5 days after injury.
53. Assess for rebleeding, change in the size of the area, presence of bright red blood, signs of increased intraocular pressure (pain, nausea and vomiting, increased inflammation), and side effects from medications.
54. Irrigate immediately with water or saline solution. For a mild burn use at least 2 L of fluid for 30 minutes; for a severe burn, use at least 10 L for 2 to 4 hours.
55. T
56. F
57. F
58. T
59. F
60. F
61. T
62. T
63. b
64. d
65. a
66. c
67. Refer to Box 31-4; there are 10 risk factors listed.
68. auditory brainstem response; evoked otoacoustic emissions test
69. Have child use hearing aid if he has one; look at the child when speaking; speak clearly and slightly slower;

eliminate background noise; use visual aids
70. T
71. F
72. T
73. F
74. T
75. T
76. 10–12 months
77. 18 months
78. two years
79. Pitch and intonation; articulation; fluency
80. Describe any activities to the child; expand on what the child says; add new information; build the child's vocabulary; repeat the child's words using adult pronunciations.
81. T
82. F
83. T
84. T

Review Questions
1. b
2. a
3. a, b, d
4. b
5. c
6. a
7. b
8. c
9. d
10. d
11. d
12. a
13. a
14. b
15. a, c, d